Emna Ellouz
Imen Ketata

Aceruloplasminemia Clinical signs and pathophysiological mechanisms

Emna Ellouz
Imen Ketata

Aceruloplasminemia Clinical signs and pathophysiological mechanisms

ScienciaScripts

Imprint

Any brand names and product names mentioned in this book are subject to trademark, brand or patent protection and are trademarks or registered trademarks of their respective holders. The use of brand names, product names, common names, trade names, product descriptions etc. even without a particular marking in this work is in no way to be construed to mean that such names may be regarded as unrestricted in respect of trademark and brand protection legislation and could thus be used by anyone.

Cover image: www.ingimage.com

This book is a translation from the original published under ISBN 978-620-6-70966-4.

Publisher:
Sciencia Scripts
is a trademark of
Dodo Books Indian Ocean Ltd. and OmniScriptum S.R.L publishing group

120 High Road, East Finchley, London, N2 9ED, United Kingdom
Str. Armeneasca 28/1, office 1, Chisinau MD-2012, Republic of Moldova, Europe
Printed at: see last page
ISBN: 978-620-7-62434-8

Aceruloplasminemia: clinical signs and pathophysiological mechanisms

Table of contents

1. Introduction

Aceruloplasminemia (ACP) is an autosomal recessive inherited disorder caused by a mutation in the ceruloplasmin (CP) gene, located on chromosome 3q23-q24 [1,2]. This mutation alters the ferroxidase activity of CP, which is crucial for the oxidation of ferrous iron to ferric iron and essential for iron incorporation into transferrin [3]. As a result, CP deficiency leads to iron deposits in many tissues, particularly the brain and liver [3]. PCA, a form of neurodegeneration with brain iron accumulation (NBIA), is a relatively rare neurodegenerative disease affecting one in every 2,000,000 people worldwide [3]. The disease generally appears in adulthood. Affected individuals often suffer from diabetes and microcytic anemia [3]. Clinical signs also include a range of neurological, psychiatric, ophthalmic and hepatic symptoms. Nevertheless, a subset of patients may initially present with neuropsychiatric (NP) symptoms without the subsequent development of diabetes or anemia. The absence of specific symptoms makes diagnosis of PCA difficult [3]. The identification of iron overload (IO) in the gray nuclei of the brain by magnetic resonance imaging (MRI) is a suggestive feature of PCA. However, the precise pathological mechanism behind this accumulation remains poorly elucidated. Biochemical analyses may reveal elevated ferritin levels, decreased serum iron and copper levels, and reduced transferrin (TS) saturation. Iron chelators are often used to treat this condition, but unfortunately, in many cases PCA is fatal [3]. Faced with clinical manifestations that show a gradual progression and the paucity of studies on PCA, we aim, through this systemic review and meta-analysis, to elucidate and explain the variations in initial clinical presentations in patients, the evolution of symptoms over the course of the disease and the emergence of cerebral iron overload (CFS). In addition, we aim to identify potential correlations between neuropsychiatric symptoms and cerebral iron overload, and to suggest alternative explanations for these symptoms.

2. Materials and methods

2.1 Study design and research strategy

We conducted a systematic review and meta-analysis in accordance with the 2020 PRISMA (Preferred Reporting Items for Systematic Reviews and MetaAnalyses) guidelines [4]. We searched PubMed and Europe PMC databases, as well as Google Scholar and Science Direct, for case reports, case series, letters to the editor, editorials and short communications relating to PCA. We included published articles and accepted manuscripts. MeSH terms were selected from the HeTOP website (https://www.hetop.eu/hetop/), and the terms selected were "aceruloplasminemia", "familial apoceruloplasmin deficiency", "ceruloplasmin deficiency", "hereditary hypoceruloplasminemia", and "hypoceruloplasminemia". We also used the following keywords: "ceruloplasmin gene", "genetic iron overload". Search terms were linked using the Boolean search operator "OR". The search syntax for collecting bibliographic data was adapted for each database and web search where appropriate: aceruloplasminemia OR "familial apoceruloplasmin deficiency" OR "hereditary hypoceruloplasminemia" OR hypoceruloplasminemia OR "ceruloplasmin deficiency" OR "ceruloplasmin gene" OR "genetic iron overload". We used an advanced search adapted for each database and Web search to select the type of publication (case reports, case series, short communications, editorials, letters to the editor). No publication date limit was set for the articles included. The last search was carried out in July 2023. To identify duplicates, all articles were imported into Mendeley. The selection of articles according to eligibility criteria was carried out in two stages. Two authors independently reviewed eligibility based on titles and abstracts using Rayyan software (https://www.rayyan.ai/). The next step was to review full-text articles for eligibility. In addition, literature review references were also examined to identify further cases [5-8].

2.2 Eligibility criteria

We included all case reports, case series, letters to the editor, short communications and editorials in which: (a) the data in the article were fully accessible; (b) the diagnosis of PCA was confirmed either by a genetic study or by low CP and brain MRI findings; (c) English was used; (d) the available data included patient demographics, their medical history, age of onset, systemic signs (diabetes, anemia, liver balance disorders), NP symptoms and additional investigations. Non-free full-text articles, poorly documented cases, case series without primary data, or pooled analyses without description of individual patient data were excluded.

2.3 Data extraction

Researchers manually collected the following information from eligible reports: article title, first author, year of publication, patient origin, patient demographics, medical history, gender, age, age at disease diagnosis, age of onset of systemic signs and NP symptoms, clinical features, liver balance disorders (elevated transaminases), results of complementary examinations and genetic studies.

2.4 Assessing the risk of bias

To assess the quality of the included articles, the Joanna Briggs Institute (JBI) Case Report Critical Appraisal Instrument was applied. The checklist includes eight questions assessing different aspects of each case report, such as patient demographics, medical history, current clinical features, details of diagnosis, treatment, post-intervention status, adverse events and lessons learned. A case report was considered acceptable if it met 5 of the 8 criteria, making it eligible for systematic review. The evaluation was carried out by two independent reviewers.

2.5 Data analysis and interpretation

We used SPSS software, developed by IBM, version 26.0 for data entry and analysis. We combined quantitative value units into a single unit: blood glucose (mmol/l), serum iron (µg/dl), ferritin (ng/ml), copper (µg/dl), CP (g/l), triglycerides (TG) (mmol/l), total cholesterol (TC) (mmol/l). Categorical variables were described using percentages and frequencies. To confirm normal distribution, we applied tests such as the Kolmogorov-Smirnov test (sample size > 50 cases) or the Shapiro-Wilk test (sample size ≤ 50 cases), as well as the moustache box and Quantil-Quantil diagram. Where data were not normally distributed, we used the median (interquartile range), otherwise we used the mean, standard deviation and extremes. For categorical variables, we used either the chi-square test or Fisher's exact test in independent samples, respecting the conditions of application of each test. To explore relationships, we calculated the unadjusted odds ratio (OR) and adjusted odds ratio (aOR) with 95% confidence intervals [95% CI] using binary or multinomial logistic regression. To compare quantitative values, when data were not normally distributed, we used the Mann-Whitney test to compare medians. However, if the distribution was normal, the t-Student test for independent samples was used to compare means. Statistical significance was determined at $p < 0.05$.

3. Results

3.1 Study features

After reviewing initial literature searches from a variety of sources (databases: 299, Internet searches: 322, and references from other journals: 4), we identified 83 articles encompassing 110 patients meeting the inclusion criteria [7-89]. The results of our literature search and selection process are summarized in **Fig. A.1.**

3.2 Risk of bias in included articles

The mean JBI bias score was 6.29/8. Among the articles included, the scores were as follows: 5 in 40 articles, 7 in 10 articles, 8 in 27 articles and 6 in 6 articles. All reports provided clear details of patient demographics, thus satisfying the first criterion. With regard to the second and third criteria, patient history and current clinical status were present in all 83 articles.

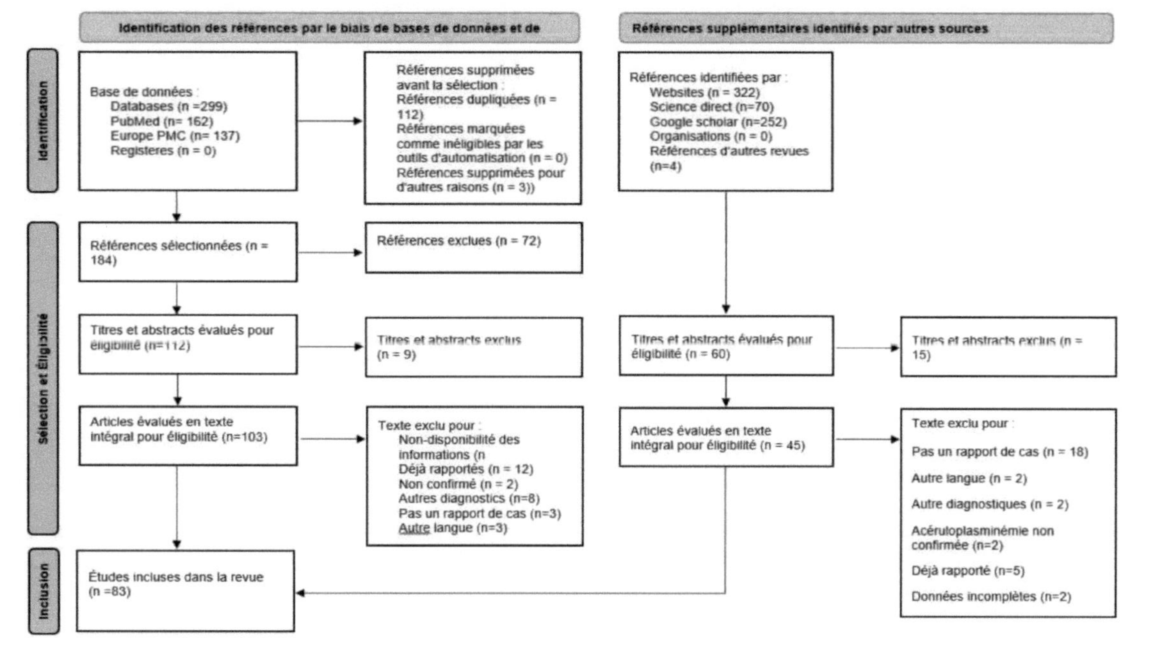

Fig. A.1 : Diagramme de PRISMA 2020 démontrant la sélection des informations à travers les différentes étapes d'une revue systématique et d'une méta-analyse.

Diagnostic tests or evaluation methods were available in all articles, thus fulfilling the fourth criterion. Genetic studies confirmed the diagnosis in 59 articles, in the remaining 24 articles the diagnosis was confirmed on CP levels and brain MRI findings. Details of treatment were available in 42 articles, while detailed explanations of post-procedure clinical states and adverse events appeared in 37 articles. Lessons learned were reported in 75 articles.

3.3 Patient demographics

The patients originated from 24 different countries, the

Japan (n = 41/110, 37.3%), Italy (n = 15/110, 13.6%) and the USA (n = 13/110, 11.8%) had the highest prevalence **(Fig. B.1).** Of 110 cases, 56 (50.9%) were women.

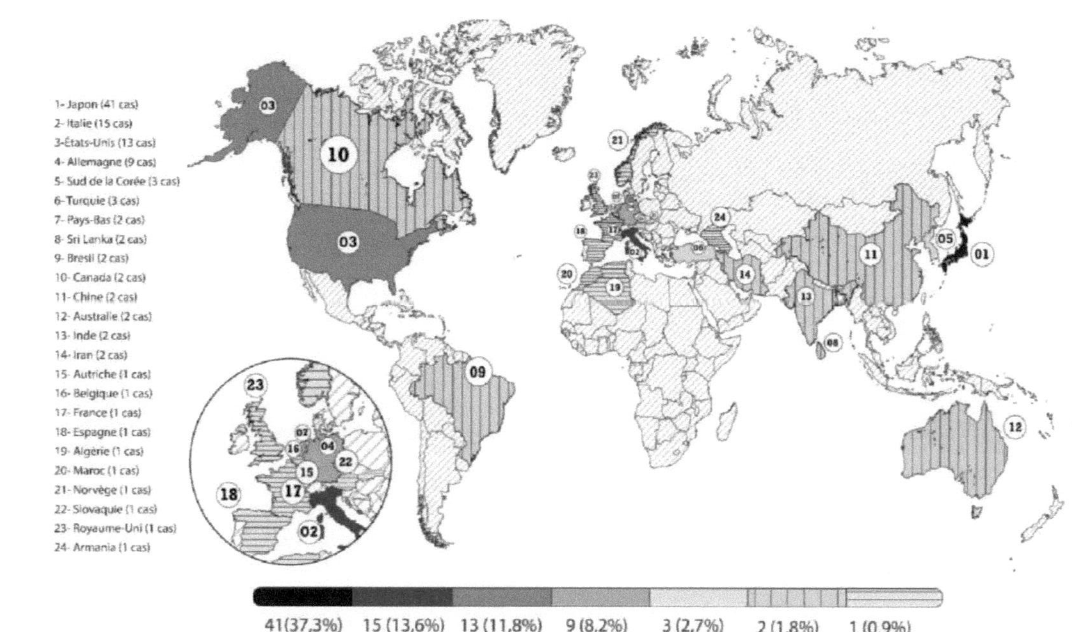

Fig. B.1 : répartition des patients ACP selon l'origine géographique

3.4 Initial clinical signs

The most frequent clinical signs at disease onset were diabetes (n = 51, 46.4%) and anemia (n = 30, 27.3%) **(Fig. B.2).** On the other hand, diabetes was not associated with pancreatic FS (p = 0.7). **Fig. B.3** summarizes the different ages of onset of the first clinical/biological signs and age at disease diagnosis.

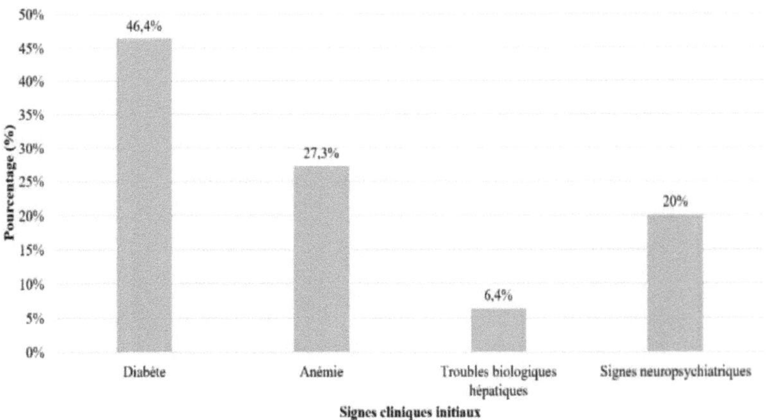

Fig. B.2: Frequency of initial clinical signs of the disease

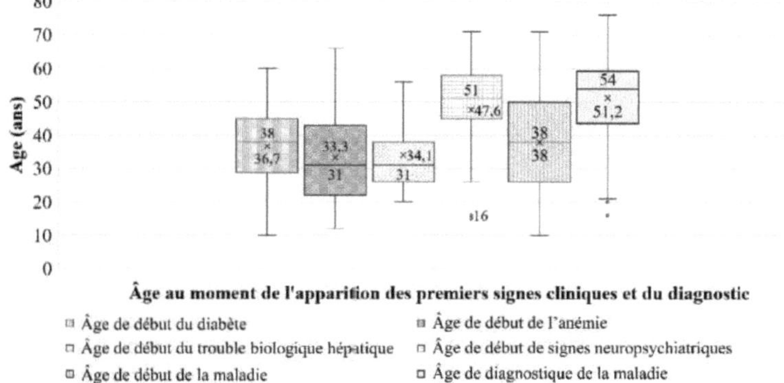

Fig. B.3: Age of onset of varicus clinical signs of the disease and age of diagnosis of PCA. The age at disease diagnosis was close to the age of onset of neuropsychiatric symptoms, while the ages of onset of diabetes, anemia and liver disorders were close. On the other hand, they were younger than the age at disease diagnosis.

In terms of initial clinical signs, diabetes was observed to be significantly more frequent in men (n = 31/54 (57.4%) vs n = 20/56 (36%), p = 0.013, OR= 2.65 [95% CI= 1,2-5.7]), while anemia was significantly the most frequent initial clinical sign in women (n = 23/56 (41.1%) vs. n = 7/54 (13%), p = 0.001, (OR=4.68 [95% CI= 1.8-12.17]) **(Fig. B.4).**

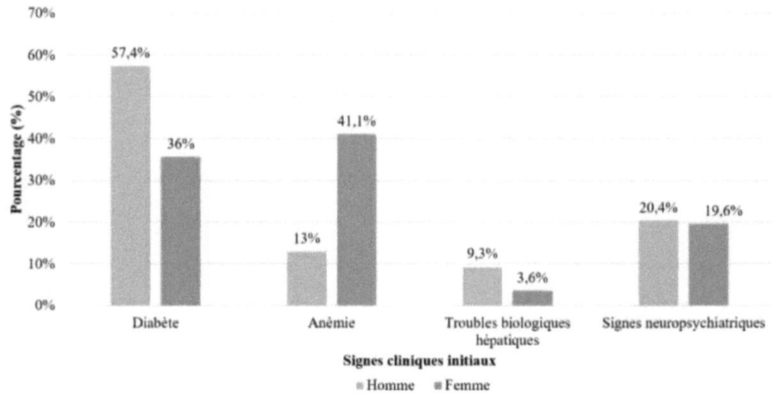

Fig. B.4: Frequency of initial clinical signs according to sex

No significant gender differences were observed for NP symptoms (p = 0.26) or liver abnormalities (p = 0.92). Men started developing diabetes 7 years earlier than women (36 (range: 24-42 years) vs. 43 (range: 3251 years), p = 0.006) **(Fig. B.5).** There was no significant difference between the 2 sexes for age of onset of anemia (p = 0.74), liver biology disorders (p = 1) and NP symptoms (p = 0.093), or for age of PCA diagnosis (p = 0.11).

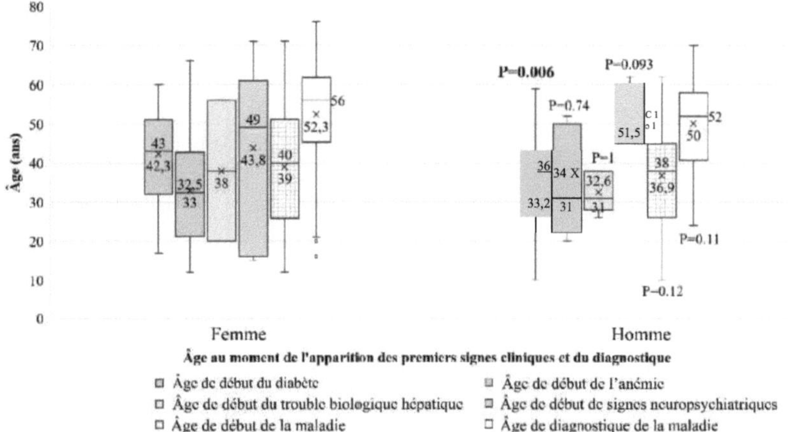

Fig. B.5: The age of onset of initial clinical/biological signs shows that the median age of onset of diabetes was younger in men and older in women. The median ages of the other signs were similar.

Consanguineous patients were 5.7 times more likely to start the disease with systemic signs (p = 0.033, OR=5.7 [95% CI=1.15-28.7]). In particular, they were 3.5 times more likely to present diabetes as their first clinical manifestation (p = 0.015, OR=3.5 [95% CI=1.26-9.4]).

(Table A.1).

Table A.1: Initial clinical/biological signs as a function of consanguinity, mutation type, sex and age at onset of disease

	Anémie			Diabète			Troubles biologiques hépatiques			Signes neuropsychiatriques		
	Résultats (n,%)	p	OR [95% IC]	Résultats (n,%)	p	OR [95% IC]	Résultats (n,%)	p	OR [95% IC]	Résultats (n,%)	p	OR [95% IC]
Consanguinité[a]												
Tous les patients (N)	26 (49.1)	0.5	1[§§]	10 (31.3)	0.015[§]	1[§§]	2 (47)	1	1[§§]	30 (53.6)	0.033[§]	1[§§]
Tous les patients (O)	6 (40)		0.7 [0.2-2.2]	22 (61.1)		3.5 [1.26-9.4]	2 (50)		1.1 [0.15-8.5]	2 (16.7)		0.17 [0.03-0.8]
Age de début de la maladie												
<30 ans												
Tous les patients (N)	19 (23.8)	0.095	1[§§]	18 (30)	0.64	1[§§]	29 (28.2)	1	1[§§]	27 (30.7)	0.24	1[§§]
Tous les patients (O)	12 (40)		2.1 [0.8-5.2]	13 (26)		0,82 [0,35-1,8]	2 (28.6)		1 [0.18-5.5]	4 (18.2)		0.5 [0.15-1.
H (O)	3 (20)	0.046[§]	1[§§]	11 (73.3)	0.002[§]	19.2 [2.9-125.1]	1 (6.7)	1	1[§§]	PP	0.1	-
F (O)	9 (56.3)		5.14 [1-25.6]	2 (12.5)		1[§§]	1 (6.3)		0.93 [0.05-16.3]	4 (25%)		-
30-50 ans												
Tous les patients (N)	38 (47.5)	0.2	1[§§]	20 (33.3)	0.018[§]	1[§§]	44 (42.7)	0.5	1[§§]	48 (54.5)	0.09	1[§§]
Tous les patients (O)	10 (33.3)		0.5 [0.2-1.3]	28 (56)		2,5 [1.2-5.5]	4 (57.1)		1.7 [0.4-8.4]	6 (27.3)		0.4 [0.14-1.14]
H (O)	2 (10)	0.008[§]	1[§§]	19 (63.3)	0.2	1	4 (13.8)	0.14	-	4 (13.8)	0.74	1[§§]
F (O)	8 (42.1)		9.8 [1.8-53.7]	9 (47.4)		0.47 [0.14-1.5]	PP		-	2 (10.5)		0.74 [0.12-4.4]

Table A.1 (continued)

	Anémie			Diabète			Troubles biologiques hépatiques			Signes neurpsychiatriques		
	Résultats (n,%)	p	OR [95% IC]	Résultats (n,%)	p	OR [95% IC]	Résultats (n,%)	p	OR [95% IC]	Résultats (n,%)	p	OR [95% IC]
30-50 ans												
Tous les patients (N)	38 (47.5)	0.2	1[§§]	20 (33.3)	0.018[§]	1[§§]	44 (42.7)	0.5	1[§§]	48 (54.5)	0.09	1[§§]
Tous les patients (O)	10 (33.3)		0.5 [0.2-1.3]	28 (56)		2,5 [1.2-5.5]	4 (57.1)		1.7 [0.4 - 8.4]	6 (27.3)		0.4 [0.14-1.14]
H (O)	2 (10)	0.008[§]	1[§§]	19 (63.3)	0.2	1	4 (13.8)	0.14	-	4 (13.8)	0.74	1[§§]
F (O)	8 (42.1)		9.8 [1.8-53.7]	9 (47.4)		0.47 [0.14-1.5]	PP		-	2 (10.5)		0.74 [0.12-4.4]
> 50 ans												
Tous les patients (N)	23 (28.7)	0.8	1[§§]	22 (36.7)	0.03[§]	1[§§]	30 (29.1)	0.67	1[§§]	19 (21.6)	0.003[§]	1[§§]
Tous les patients (O)	8 (26.7)		0.9 [0.35-2.3]	9 (18)		0.4 [0.1-0.9]	1 (14.3)		0.4 [0.05-3.5]	12 (54.5)		4.3 [1.6-11.6]
H (O)	2 (20)	1	1[§§]	1 (11.1)	0.13	1[§§]	PP	1	-	7 (70)	0.02[§]	7.5 [1,4-40.2]
F (O)	6 (28.6)		1.6 [0.25-9.8]	8 (38.1)		5.5 [0.6-52.3]	1 (4.8)		-	5 (23.8)		1[§§]
Mutation[**]												
Hétérozygote(O) /HC (O)	PP/6 (40)	0.5	1[§§]	PP/5 (3.33)	0.03[§]	1[§§]	PP/1 (6.7)	0.9	1[§§]	7 (100)/ 3 (20)	0.001[§]	1[§§]
Homozygotes (O)	22 (34.4)		0.76 [0.2-2]	32 (50)		3.4 [1.1-10.3]	3 (4.7)		1 [0.1-10.4]	6 (9.4)		0.12 [0.03-0.4]

*Disponible dans 68 cas; ** Disponible dans 86 cas (64 homozygotes, 7 hétérozygotes, 15 hétérozygotes composites); OR, odds ratio non ajusté; IC, intervalle de confiance; F, femme; H, Homme; N, patients sans symptômes; O, patients avec symptômes; HC, hétérozygotes composites; PP, pas de patient; § signification statistique à p<0.05; §§ Références.

Before the age of 30, women were more likely to have anemia (56.3% vs. 20%, p = 0.046, OR=5.14 [95% CI=1-25.6]), while men were more predisposed to diabetes (73.3% vs. 12.5%, p = 0.002, OR=19.2 [95% CI= 2.9-125.1]). Between the ages of 30 and 50, the risk of anemia was also significantly higher in women, where the risk was multiplied by 4.66 (p = 0.008, OR=9.8 [95% IC=1.8-53.7]). This age group was associated with diabetes irrespective of gender (56% vs. 33.3%, p = 0.018, OR=2.5 [95% CI=1.2-5.5]). Furthermore, NP symptoms were highly significant in patients aged over 50 (54.5% vs. 21.6%, p = 0.003, OR = 4.3 [95% CI = 1.6-11.6]). Male gender was also associated with a higher risk of developing NP symptoms after the age of 50 (p = 0.02, OR=7.5 [95% CI=1.4-40.2]). On the other hand, diabetes was negatively associated with patients aged 50 and over (p = 0.03, OR=0.4 [95% CI=0.1-0.9]). Patients who had started diabetes had a ferritin level ≥ 700 ng/ml (ferritin available in 91/110 cases) more often than patients who had not started diabetes (40/47

(85.1%) vs. 25/44 (56.8%), p = 0.004, OR= 4.34 [95% CI= 1.6-11.8]). We also found that ferritin < 700 ng/ml was more frequent in patients starting with anemia than in patients without anemia (14/24 (58.3%) vs. 12/67 (17.9%), p < 0.001, OR= 6.4 [95% CI= 2.317.8]). Similarly, a serum copper level ≤ 40 µg/dl (serum copper available in 72/110 cases) was observed more frequently in patients who started with diabetes (37/38 (97.4%) vs. 27/34 (79.4%), p = 0.04, OR= 9,6 [95% IC= 1.1-82.6]). On the other hand, iron levels showed no association with the onset of diabetes (p = 0.5) or anemia (p = 0.3), and copper was not associated with the onset of anemia (p = 1).

Multivariate analysis revealed that male sex (p = 0.04, aOR=3.6 [95% CI=1-12.2]), ferritin ≥ 700 ng/ml (p = 0.01, aOR=12.32 [95% CI=1.8-82.4]) and consanguinity (p = 0.046, aOR=6 [95% CI= 1.35-35.4]) were significantly associated with diabetes. Anemia remained significantly associated with female gender (p = 0.005, aOR=6.5 [95% CI=1.7-23.8]) and ferritin<700 ng/ml (p = 0.004, aOR=5.7 [95% CI=1.7-19]). Only consanguinity was inversely associated with NP symptoms (p = 0.04, aOR=0.2 [95% CI=0.03-0.9]). **Fig. C.**1 summarizes the initial clinical/biological signs according to age of disease onset, and shows the predictive factor for each sign.

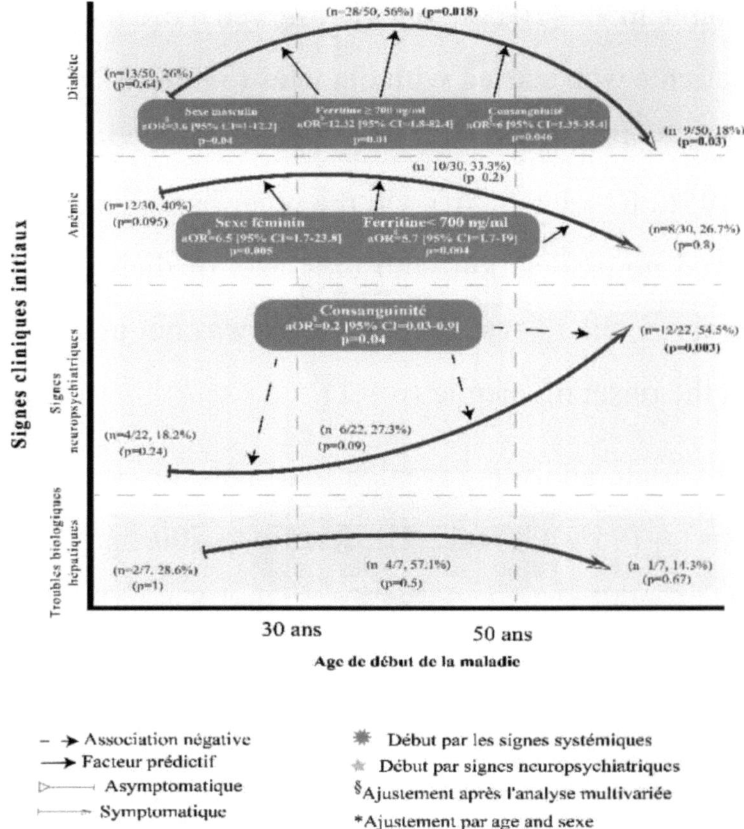

Fig. C.1: Initial clinical signs according to age of onset and risk factors for their appearance

3.4 Clinical signs during follow-up

Among patients with systemic disease onset, 63/88 (71.6%) developed NP symptoms after a median delay of 13.5 years (range: 4-24.25 years). Among these patients, the median age of onset of NP symptoms during follow-up was 52 years (range: 48-57 years). After adjustment for gender and consanguinity, while NP symptoms during follow-up were negatively associated with patients aged under 30 (p=0.027, aOR=0.5 [95% CI=0.004-0.72]) and between 30 and 50 (p=0.04, aOR=0.23 [95% CI=0.06-0.9]), they were positively associated with patients aged 50 or over (p=0.002, aOR=10 [95% CI=2.4-43]). Of the 22 patients with NP symptoms at onset, 6 (27.3%) developed anemia and 4 (18.2%) diabetes, with a median delay of 2 (range: 0.5-6 years) and 1 (range: 0.75-18.5 years) respectively. Furthermore, after adjustment for consanguinity, gender and age, presentation of NP symptoms as initial clinical signs remained negatively associated with diabetes and anemia during follow-up (p < 0.001, aOR=0.024 [95% CI=0.003-0.18], p = 0.008, aOR=0. 1 [95% CI=0.021-0.5] respectively). The presentation of systemic signs at the start of the disease and consanguinity were both predictive of the appearance of NP symptoms during follow-up (p = 0.033, aOR=15.16 [95% IC= 1.2-195], p = 0.04, aOR=4.5 [95% IC=1-20.1] respectively). **Fig. C.2** summarizes the evolution of clinical signs during patient follow-up as a function of patient age and different predictive factors.

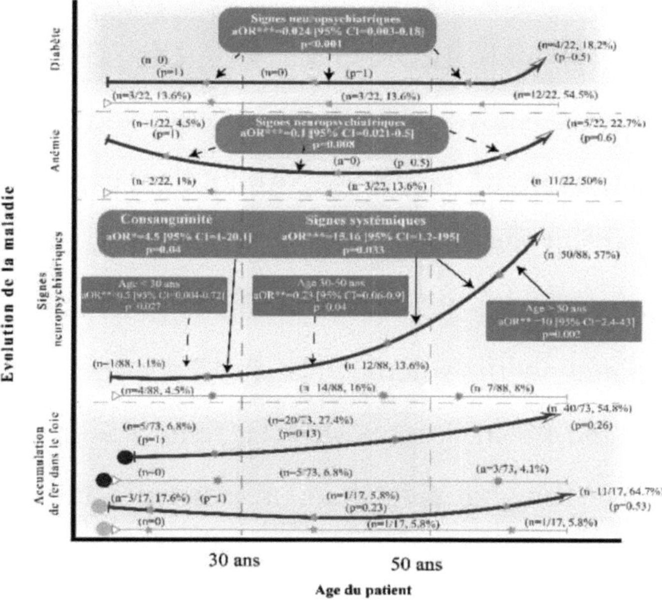

● Parmi 88 patients débutant par les signes systémiques, l'exploration abdominale était disponibles dans 73 cas

● Parmi 22 patients débutant par les signes neuropsychiatriques, l'exploration abdominale était disponibles dans 17 cas

**Ajustement selon le sexe et la consanguinité

***Ajustement selon l'âge, le sexe et la consanguinité

Fig. C.2: Evolution of clinical signs during follow-up as a function of patient age and various predictive factors

3.6. Disease characteristics

Median age at diagnosis was significantly higher than age at onset of anemia, diabetes, liver disorders and NP symptoms (p < 0.001, p < 0.01, p = 0.001, p < 0.01 respectively). Diabetes appeared significantly earlier in men than in women (p < 0001). The prevalence of dystonia was significantly higher in women (p = 0.014, OR=3.92 [95% CI=1.3-11.63]). **Table B.1** shows the demographic and clinical characteristics of the disease. Abdominal exploration was carried out in 90 patients. It revealed isolated hepatic FS in 68 cases (75.5%), hepatic FS associated with splenic FS in 3 cases (3.3%), pancreatic FS in 8 cases (8.9%), renal FS in 1 case (1.1%). Ten patients had a normal abdominal examination (11.1%). Pancreatic FS was not associated with diabetes (p = 0.7). Similarly, hepatic FS showed no association with diabetes or anemia (p = 0.1, p = 0.4 respectively).

Table B.1: Disease characteristics

	All patients	Hommee[i]	Woman	P	OR [95% CI]
Age at onset of disease (years)	37.9 ± 13.9 [10-71]	36.8 ± 12,15 [10-62]	39 ± 15,53 [12-71]	0,36	-
Age at diagnosis of illness (years)	54 (range: 43.75-59.25)	52 (range: 45-56)	56 (range: 45.25-61.7)	0.49	-
Age at onset of anemia (years)	50 (range: 29-56)	50 (range: 29.5-56)	49 (range: 25-56)	0.89	-
Age at onset of diabetes (years)	41.87 ± 14.2 [10-72]	38 (range: 26-42.7)	50 (range: 38-60)	<0.001 §	-
Age of onset of biological disorders liver (years)	36.5 (range: 30.25-50.5)	35 (range: 30-38)	51 (range: 27-62)	0.29	-
Age at onset of disorders neurological/psychiatric (years)	50.5 ± 12.67 [15-75]	50 (range: 45-56)	55 (range: 48-61)	0.09	-
Isolated systemic signs	25 (22.7%)	13 (24.1%)	12 (21.4%)	0.7	-
Isolated neurological symptoms	10 (9.1%)	6 (11.1%)	4 (7.1%)	0.47	-
Isolated psychiatric symptoms	1 (0.9%)	1 (1.9%)	PP	-	-
Neurological and psychiatric signs	5 (4.5%)	3 (5.6%)	2 (3.6%)	0.23	-
Neurological and systemic signs	42 (38.2%)	19 (35.2%)	23 (41.1%)	0.62	-
Psychiatric and systemic signs	3 (2.7%)	PP	3 (5.4%)	-	-
Neurological, psychiatric and systemic	24 (21.8%)	12 (22.2%)	12 (21.4%)	0.92	-
Systemic signs	93 (34.5%)	44 (81.5%)	49 (87.5%)	0.38	1.59 [0.55-4.53]
Diabetes	69 (62.7%)	34 (63%)	35 (62.5%)	0.96	0.98 [0.45-2.12]
Type 1	18 (25.3%)	13 (37.1%)	5 (13.9%)	0,021 §	0.25 [0.07-0.81
Type 2*	53 (74.6%)	22 (62.8%)	31 (86.1%)	0.021 §	1.23 [1.23-12.7]
Not checked**	14 (73.7%)	9 (100%)	5 (50%)	0.033§	-
Glucose intolerance	4 (3.6%)	1 (1.9%)	3 (5.4%)	0.34	3 [0.3-29.7]
Anemia	74	28	46	0.001 §	1.23 [1.23-

29

| | (67.3%) | (51.9%) | (82.1%) | | 12.7] |
| Uncontrolled[1] | 15 (100%) | 6 (100%) | 9 (100%) | - | - |

Table B.1 (continued)

	All patients	Hommee[i]	Woman	P	OR [95% CI]
Neurological symptoms					
Symptomatic	82 (74.5%)	40 (74.1%)	42 (75%)	0.91	0.95 [0.4-2.23]
Asymptomatic	28 (25.5%)	14 (25.9%)	14 (25%)	-	-
Cognitive disorders	52 (47.3%)	26 (48.1%)	26 (46.4%)	0.85	0.9 [0.4-1.97]
Ataxia	42 (38.2%)	21 (38.9%)	20 (37%)	0.88	0.94 [0.43-2.03
Parkinsonism	23 (21%)	10 (18.5%)	13 (23.2%)	0.56	1.3 [0.5-3.19]
Abnormal movements	38 (34.5%)	15 (27.7%)	23 (41.1%)	0.09	2 [0.8-4.47]
Dystonia	21 (19.1%)	5 (9.3%)	16 (28.6%)	0.014§	3.92 [1.3-11.63
Blepharospasm	8 (7.3%)	1 (1.9%)	7 (12.5%)	-	-
Cervical and mandibular	5 (4.5%)	1 (1.9%)	4 (7.1%)	-	-
Langual	1 (0.9%)	PP	1 (1.8%)	-	-
Lower limb	1 (0.9%)	PP	1 (1.8%)	-	-
Missing	6 (5.4%)	2 (3.7%)	4 (7.1%)	-	-
Oral dyskinesia	14 (12.7%)	6 (11.1%)	8 (14.3%)	-	-
Choreography	9 (8.2%)	2 (3.7%)	7 (12.5%)	-	-
Chorea-athetosis	2 (1.8%)	1 (1.9%)	1 (1.8%)	-	-
Myoclonus	2 (1.8%)	1 (1.9%)	PP	-	-
Trembling	4 (3.6%)	1 (1.9%)	3 (5.3%)	-	-
Akathisie	1 (0.9%)	1 (1.9%)	PP	-	-
Hyperkinesia	1 (0.9%)	PP	1 (1.8%)	-	-
Dysarthria	25 (22.7%)	14 (25.9%)	11 (19.6%)	0.43	0.7 [0.28-1.7]
Vertigo	5 (4.5%)	1 (1.9%)	4 (7.1%)	-	-
Epileptic seizure	4 (3.6%)	2 (3.7%)	2 (3.6%)	-	-
Swallowing disorders	4 (3.6%)	2 (3.7%)	2 (3.6%)	-	-
Frontal lobe syndrome	3 (2.7%)	2 (3.7%)	1 (1.8%)	-	-
Consciousness disorders	2 (1.8%)	2 (3.7%)	PP	-	-
Lower limb heaviness	2 (1.8%)	2 (3.7%)	PP	-	-

Table B.1 (continued)

	All patients	Hommee[i]	Woman	P	OR [95% CI]
Psychiatric symptoms					
Symptomatic	30 (27.3%)	14 (25.9%)	16 (28.6%)	0.7	1.1 [0.5-2.6]
Asymptomatic	80 (72.7%)	40 (74.1%)	40 (71.4%)	-	-
Behavioural problems (aggressiveness	15 (13.6%)	7 (13%)	8 (14.3%)	0.84	1.19 [0.37-3.3]
Depression	12 (10.9%)	7 (13%)	5 (8.9%)	0.5	0.65 [0.19-2.2]
Anxiety	6 (5.5)	PP	6 (10.7%)	0.027§	-
Apathy	5 (4.5)	3 (5.6%)	2 (3.6%)	0.62	0.63 [0.1-3.9]
Hallucination	2 (1.8%)	1 (1.9%)	1 (1.8%)	0.97	0.96 [0.05 15.8]
Bipolar disorder	2 (1.8%)	PP	2 (3.6%)	0.49	-
Schizophrenia-like psychosis	1 (0.9%)	1 (1.9%)	PP	0.6	-
Other clinical signs					
Asthenia	15 (13.6%)	6 (11.1%)	9 (16.1%)	-	-
Hearing loss	3 (2.7%)	2 (3.7%)	1 (1.8%)	-	-
Muscle cramps	2 (1.8%)	2 (3.7%)	PP	-	-
Nyctalopia	1 (0.9%)	1 (1.9%)	PP	-	-
Paroxysmal febrile peak (/6 months)	1 (0.9%)	1 (1.9%)	PP	-	-

*Type of diabetes available in 71 cases (35 men and 36 women); **available in 19 cases (9 men and 10 women); ↑ available in 15 cases (6 men and 9 women); J reference; PP, no patient; § statistically significant at p<0.05.

Hemoglobin levels were significantly lower in women than in men (p = 0.001), and HbA1c and ferritin levels higher in men (p = 0.039 and p = 0.028 respectively) **(Table C.1).** Median blood glucose levels were significantly lower in patients with epileptic seizures than in those without (1.8 mmol/l vs. 8.3 mmol/l, p = 0.019). **Table D.1** summarizes brain MRI findings and the association between NP symptoms and CFS. Exclusive correlations were observed between abnormal movements and FS of the putamen and pallidum (p < 0.05), while cognitive impairment showed an association with FS of the cerebral cortex (p < 0.05).

Table C.1: Biological results

	Normal range	Results	p
			0.001 | |
Hb (g/dl)*	H ≥13	H 11.5 (9.9-13)	| |
	F ≥12	F 9.8 (9-10.6)	
Anemia		H (26, 74.3%)	0.003 | |
		F (39, 97.5%)	| |
VCM (fl)**	VCM ≥80	76.1 ± 7.6 [50-95]	
Serum iron (μg(dL)ᵗ		26 (17- 34.5)	
	H 70-175	H 26.2 (16-38)	0.19
	F 50 - 150	F 22 (17-31)	
Collapsed	H< 70	H 36 (85.7%)	
	F<50	F 39 (83%)	0.6
Ferritin (ng/mL)⁺		1111.4(540-1530)	0.028 | |
	H 18 - 270	H 1225 [835-1699]	| |
	F 18-160	F 891 [461-1499]	
High		85 (93.4%)	
Ferritin > 700 ng/ml		H 38 (86.7%)	0.002 | |
		F 27 (57.4%)	| |
Transferrin saturation (%)**		11 (6.8-13.7)	
	20 - 50	H 11.5 (8.6-17.5)	0.09
		F 9.5 (6-12)	
Bottom	< 20	34 (87.2%)	
Plasma copper levels (μg(dL)	70 -140	9 (5.2-16.5)	
		H 8 (5.2-15.2)	0.4
		F 9.4 (5.2-19.6)	
Bottom	< 70	73 (100%)	
Serum ceruloplasmin (g/l)¹	0.2 - 0.6	0.01 (0-0.2)	
		H 0.006 (0-0.02)	0.8
		F 0.0 (0-0.023)	
		HM 0.0005 (0-0.02)	-
		HC 0.026 (0-0.075)	<0.001 IIII
		HZ 0.11 (0.1-0.11)	<0.001 II
Bottom	< 0.2	108 (99%)	
Liver function¹¹			
ALT (U/L)	7 - 55	25 (17-54)	
High		9 (20.9)	
AST (U/L)	8 - 48	23.5 (17-41.5)	
High		7 (16.3%)	
Fasting blood glucose (mmol/l)¹¹¹	<5.6	8 (5-11.8)	
		H 8.8 (5-13.9)	
		F 6.5 (4.8-9.3)	
HbAlc (%)§	< 5.7	8.5 ± 2.3 [5.3- 14.5] H 9.4 ± 2.4 [6-14.5] F 7.8 ± 1.9 [5.3-11.9]	0,039 | | | |

Hb, hemoglobin; MCV, mean corpuscular volume; ALT, alanine transaminase; AST, aspartate transaminase; HbA1c, glycated hemoglobin, H, male; F, female; HZ, heterozygotes; HM, homozygotes (reference); HC, compound heterozygotes; *available in 75 cases (35 in men, 40 in women); **available in 66 cases; !available in 89 cases (42 in men, 47 in women); Javailable in 91 cases (44 in men, 47 in women); JJavailable in 39 cases; Havailable in 72 cases; *available in 109 cases; **available in 43 cases; **'='available in 34 cases; §available in 28 cases; HH statistically significant at p<0. 05.

Table D.1: Magnetic resonance imaging findings and association with neurological symptoms

Resonance imaging Results magnetic*	(all)	Symptoms of NP[t]	Disorders At i *axe[1] cognitive[tt]		Abnormal movements "He
Normal	6 (6.2%)				
Iron overload in brain	81 (83.5%)	62 (81.6%)**	36 (83.7%)**	33 (86.8%)**	32 (88.9%)**
Nodes of the base	79 (81.1%)	61 (80.2%)**	35 (81.4%)**	32 (84.2%)**	27 (75%)**
Caudate nucleus	37 (38.1%)	27 (35.5%)**	11 (25.6%)**	16 (42.1%)**	12 (33.3%)**
Putamen	34 (35%)	29 (38.1%)**	19 (44.2%)**	13 (34.2%)**	7 (19.5%)[t]
Pallidium	9 (9.2%)	8 (10.5%)**	4 (9.3%)**	6 (15.7%)**	9 (25%)[t]
Striatium	14 (14.4%)	10 (13.1%)**	4 (9.3%)**	4 (10.5%)**	2 (5.5%)**
Cores lentiforms	10 (10.3%)	7 (9.2%)**	5 (11.6%)**	4 (10.5%)**	1 (2.7%)**
Serrated core	59 (60.8%)	44 (57.9%)**	25 (58.1%)**	25 (65.8%)**	23 (63.9%)**
Thalamus	57 (58.7%)	41 (53.9%)**	25 (58.1%)**	22 (57.9%)**	21 (58.3%)**
Medium brain	25 (25.8%)	21 (27.6%)**	17 (39.5%)**	12 (31.6%)**	11 (30.5%)
Subtantia nigra	15 (15.4%)	-	-	-	-
Red core	13 (13.4%)	-	-	-	-
Cerebellar peduncle	2 (2.06%)	-	-	-	-
Cerebral cortex	16 (16.5%)	15 (19.7%)	12 (27.9%)[t]	9 (23.7%)**	9 (25%)**
T2 hyperintensity of the white matter	9 (9.2%)	-	-	-	-
Periventricular	2 (2.06%)	-	-	-	-
U-shaped fiber	1 (1.03%)	-	-	-	-
Cerebral atrophy	16 (16.5%)	-	-	-	-
Cerebellar atrophy	5 (5.1%)	-	-	-	-
Global atrophy	5 (5.1%)	-	-	-	-
Global atrophy without iron overload	1 (1.03%)	-	-	-	-
Superficial siderosis	4 (4.1%)	-	-	-	-

*Available in 97 cases; **not statistically significant at p≥0.05; ↑ statistically significant

Figs. D.1, D.2, D.3 and D.4 summarize the predictive factors for CFS and involvement of the basal ganglia, thalamus and dentate nuclei. After adjustment for age and sex, anemia was significantly associated with mesencephalic FS (p=0.007, aOR=17.5 [95% CI=2.1-141]). After adjustment for the onset of diabetes as an initial clinical sign or during follow-up, male gender was also negatively associated with CFS (p = 0.02, aOR=0.19 [95% CI=0.5- 0.7]).

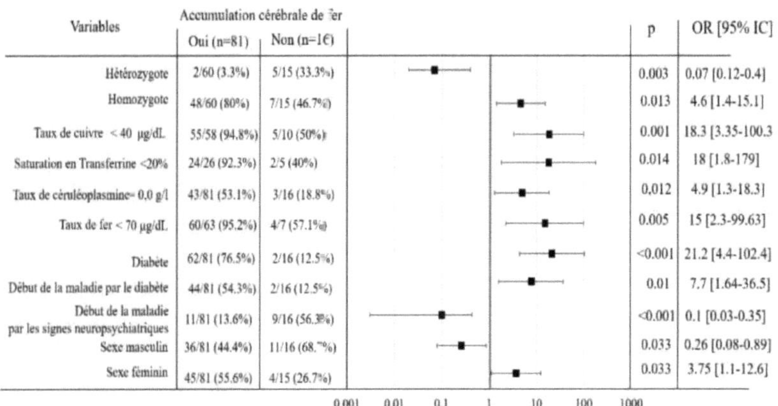

Variables	Accumulation cérébrale de fer			p	OR [95% IC]
	Oui (n=81)	Non (n=16)			
Hétérozygote	2/60 (3.3%)	5/15 (33.3%)		0.003	0.07 [0.12-0.4]
Homozygote	48/60 (80%)	7/15 (46.7%)		0.013	4.6 [1.4-15.1]
Taux de cuivre < 40 µg/dL	55/58 (94.8%)	5/10 (50%)		0.001	18.3 [3.35-100.3
Saturation en Transferrine <20%	24/26 (92.3%)	2/5 (40%)		0.014	18 [1.8-179]
Taux de céruléoplasmine= 0,0 g/l	43/81 (53.1%)	3/16 (18.8%)		0,012	4.9 [1.3-18.3]
Taux de fer < 70 µg/dL	60/63 (95.2%)	4/7 (57.1%)		0.005	15 [2.3-99.63]
Diabète	62/81 (76.5%)	2/16 (12.5%)		<0.001	21.2 [4.4-102.4]
Début de la maladie par le diabète	44/81 (54.3%)	2/16 (12.5%)		0.01	7.7 [1.64-36.5]
Début de la maladie par les signes neuropsychiatriques	11/81 (13.6%)	9/16 (56.3%)		<0.001	0.1 [0.03-0.35]
Sexe masculin	36/81 (44.4%)	11/16 (68.7%)		0.033	0.26 [0.08-0.89]
Sexe féminin	45/81 (55.6%)	4/15 (26.7%)		0.033	3.75 [1.1-12.6]

0,001   0,01   0,1   1   10   100   1000

Fig. D.1: Forest plot of predictive factors for CFS

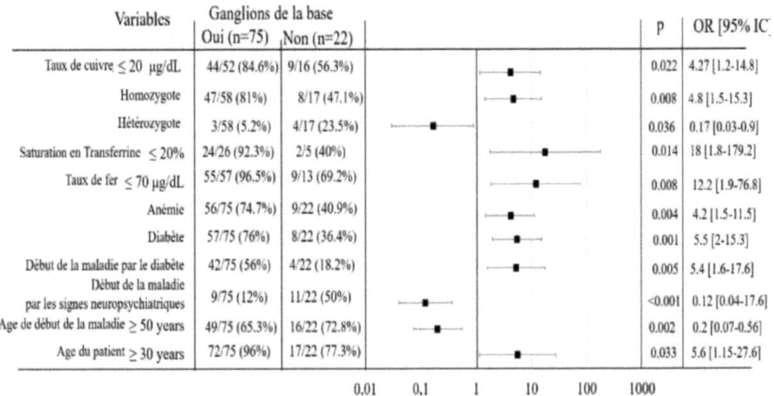

Fig. D.2: Forest plot of predictors of basal ganglia FS

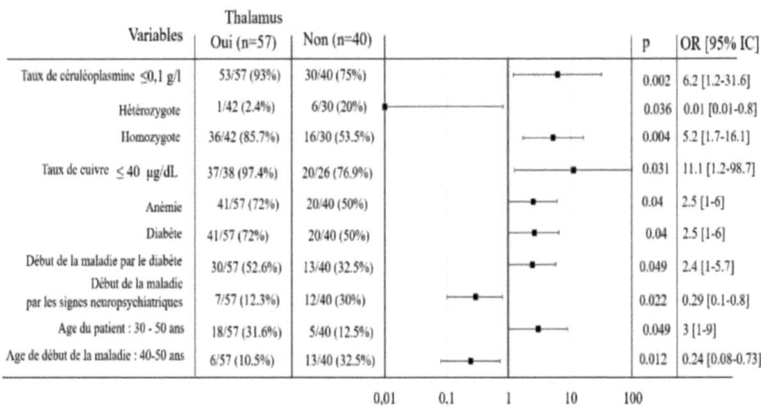

Fig. D.3: Factors associated with iron overload in the thalamus

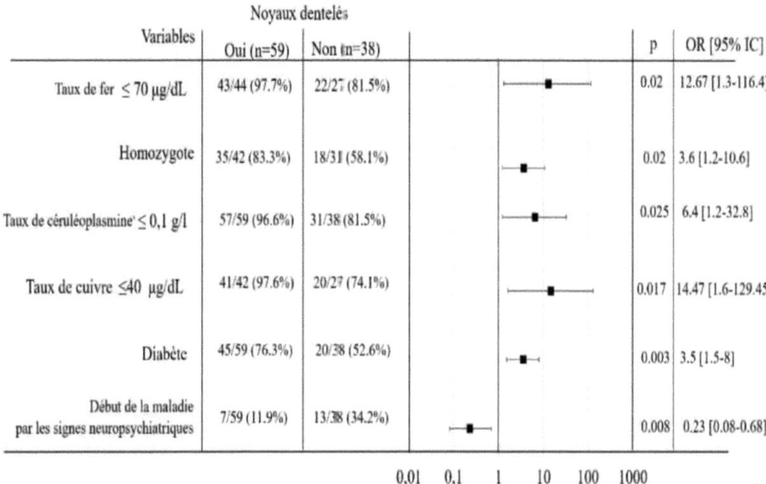

Fig. D.4: Factors associated with the SF of the serrated core

4. Discussion

To the best of our knowledge, this is the first meta-analysis and largest case series of PCA reported to date. This meta-analysis provides an update on the epidemiology of PCA worldwide, an overview of clinical symptoms, biological and radiological findings. It improves our understanding of initial clinical signs and their progression in men and women, and suggests new pathophysiological hypotheses for clinical signs and CFS. Consistent with previous literature reviews, Japan and Italy had the highest prevalence of PCA [90,91]. We found that the USA was the third country with a high frequency. This had not been reported previously.

Nevertheless, PCA has been documented in other European countries, as well as in Asia and Africa. Depending on the age of onset of the disease, anemia emerged as the main initial symptom observed in individuals under the age of 30. In patients aged between 30 and 50, diabetes was more frequent than anemia.

Conversely, NP symptoms occurred mainly in patients aged 50 and over. With the exception of the age of onset of anemia (<20 years) our result was similar to that described by Miyajima et al [92]. The median age at disease onset, diabetes onset, NP symptom onset and disease diagnosis were similar to those reported in a review including 55 patients [91]. At the same time, we found a younger median age of onset of anemia (31 years) (39.5 years) [91]. Similarly, several studies have reported a similar median age at disease diagnosis (~ 40 years) [19,91,93,94]. We observed that the median age at diagnosis was close to the median age of onset of NP symptoms. However, it was significantly older than the median age of onset of systemic signs (p < 0.001). This finding was also consistent with the findings of Vroegindeweij et al. and Bianca et al [91,94]. Our study revealed that the diagnosis of PCA is usually made after the onset of NP symptoms, whereas diagnosis based on systemic signs is less frequent. Initiation of the disease by anemia and/or diabetes presents a difficult clinical diagnostic situation [90]. Our data underline the importance of raising awareness of the disease to reduce the long delay in diagnosis of the first symptoms. Indeed, PCA requires early recognition and should not be neglected, particularly in cases of diabetes or anemia, since we identified these as the two most frequent indicators of disease onset and progression. This finding is consistent with the results of previous investigations [7,19,90,91]. Previous studies have shown that the presence of diabetes in PCA can be attributed to excessive iron overload within the pancreas [95]. Nevertheless, we found no significant correlation between the onset of diabetes or its occurrence during follow-up and FS in pancreatic tissue. We also speculate that hepatic FS may be included in the mechanism of diabetes onset, as it plays a role in glucose haemostasis and insulin sensitivity [96]. The liver interacts functionally with adipose tissue, another key regulator of energy balance that plays a fundamental role in insulin resistance, diabetes development and obesity

[97, 98]. While in our included cases, the description of obesity was not noted, the occurrence of diabetes in PCA can be elucidated by considering the influence of adipose tissue [97,98]. In fact, ceruloplasmin is produced and secreted as adipokine by adipose tissue, and adipose tissue functionality is affected by iron homeostasis [97,98].

While the precise mechanism behind the emergence of diabetes in ACP patients remains poorly understood, our meta-analysis proposes a new pathophysiological hypothesis. This implies that diabetes could potentially be linked to an irregular metabolic process involving disturbances in serum ferritin, iron and copper levels. Our results suggest that elevated ferritin levels in excess of 700 ng/ml may contribute to the early onset of diabetes. Recent reports have demonstrated an increased risk of diabetes with high serum ferritin levels in healthy individuals [99]. These findings had been supported by two other meta-analyses [19, 20]. In fact, Aregbesola et al demonstrated that in healthy individuals, ferritin concentrations ranging from 228 to 939 ng/ml were associated with an approximately 1.5-fold increased likelihood of developing diabetes [100]. In addition, several recent studies have demonstrated a high incidence of diabetes within 5 to 15 years in otherwise healthy individuals with high serum ferritin levels [99, 101]. Furthermore, we noted that remarkably low serum copper levels (<40ug/dl) emerged as an important factor associated with the onset of diabetes. This finding was corroborated by several studies that investigated the relationship between serum copper levels and the onset of diabetes in healthy individuals [102-105]. They found that disruption of copper metabolism gives rise to diabetes, both directly and indirectly, via oxidative stress, involving reactions such as the Fenton and Haber-Weiss reactions [104, 106]. This oxidative stress leads to impairment of pancreatic islet beta cells, affecting insulin secretion, contributing to peripheral insulin resistance and increasing vulnerability to diabetes [102,103]. Similarly, outside the PCA, cases of pronounced copper deficiency in the body result in insufficient synthesis of the transporter protein Glut-2, causing disruption of insulin generation [102]. On the other hand, it has been established that increased insulin levels can trigger cellular iron uptake [102]. This suggests that patients who started out with diabetes may develop iron-deficiency anemia in the PCA. Similarly, Jeppu et al. found an inverse association between serum CP levels and fasting blood glucose in patients without PCA [106]. All these findings corroborate our findings and suggest that the link between PCA and diabetes forms a vicious circle. Thus, diabetes is associated with various factors and deterioration of pancreatic tissue due to oxidative stress, rather than SF in the pancreas. Another unique finding was that men were more likely to develop the disease through diabetes and women through anemia, otherwise no significant difference had been shown for other symptoms. Ferritin has been identified as a trigger for the onset of diabetes and varied according to sex and ethnic origin [107]. Our results showed that men were more likely to have ferritin levels > 700 ng/ml than women, who more frequently had levels < 700 ng/ml. Thus, whereas we had found that a level above 700 ng/ml was associated with the onset of diabetes and a level below 700 was associated with the onset of anemia, this discrepancy leads us to propose that higher ferritin levels in men than in women could contribute to an increased susceptibility to the onset of diabetes in men and anemia in women. Our study revealed that women had lower median iron, higher serum copper and significantly reduced ferritin levels compared to men. This difference could explain the increase in anemia rather than diabetes in women. Similarly, compared with men among healthy individuals, women face additional sources of iron deficiency due to menstruation, pregnancy and breastfeeding, factors that could contribute to lower ferritin levels [108]. Further research is needed to better understand the reasons for the divergence in disease onset, with diabetes occurring predominantly in men and anemia in women.

Another interesting finding was that of the six cases included for which data on TC levels were available, 3 had elevated TC levels. At the same time, TG levels were available in three studies, with normal levels in all cases. In a ceruloplasmin-deficient mouse model, Raia et al showed a link between iron and lipid dysmetabolism [109]. In fact, their research demonstrated that treatment of these mice with ceruloplasmin limited macrophage infiltration of adipose and liver tissue, reduced serum TG levels and partially restored adipokine levels in adipose tissue. [109]. In addition, carriage of heterozygous CP variants, associated with elevated serum ferritin levels and iron deposition in the liver, has been considered a risk factor for progression to non-alcoholic fatty liver/non-alcoholic steatotic hepatitis (NAFLD/NASH) [110]. Although we found only one reported case of PCA with steatosis in our research, and no case had NAFLD/NASH [46], these findings highlight the crucial link between iron regulation and lipid metabolism. Further investigations are needed to unravel and clarify this relationship. In conjunction with the previously elucidated pathophysiological process of CFS in PCA, the current meta-analysis presents an innovative explanation. We believe that diabetes may play an indirect and crucial role. Our univariate analysis revealed evidence that diabetes represented a significant common FS risk factor for the brain, basal ganglia, thalamus and dentate nuclei. Similarly, it has been observed in recent research that brain iron levels in people with diabetes (outside PCA) were significantly higher in specific areas such as the striatum encompassing the caudate, putamen, pallidumn and frontal lobe cortex, compared with healthy individuals. [30]. Indeed, increased glucose levels can lead to the release of advanced glycation end products that can trigger inflammation and oxidative stress, potentially influencing CFS [102, 1061. In addition, oxidative stress has the potential to disrupt the integrity of the blood-brain barrier, potentially facilitating the passage of more iron into brain tissue [102,106]. Given that evidence from in vitro studies shows that insulin induces relocalization of transferrin receptors to the cell surface, leading to increased cellular iron uptake [111]. Thus, under conditions of insulin resistance, hyperinsulinemia may play a role in the circulation of soluble transferrin receptors [111]. Furthermore, elevated ferritin levels have been shown to correlate negatively with insulin sensitivity [111]. Furthermore, we found that a TS < 20% was significantly associated with CFS, suggesting a greater amount of soluble transferrin in the blood and brain in PCA. Given that PCA is characterized by high ferritin levels, poorly controlled diabetes on insulin suggesting insulin resistance, and low TS, it's clear that diabetes, through an indirect effect, may be one of multiple mechanisms for CFS in PCA. This interesting finding may help us to understand why patients who started with diabetes had a higher risk of developing CFS than other patients, and may provide an explanation for the absence or low CFS in patients who initially manifest NP symptoms and subsequently do not develop systemic signs. Further research is still needed to establish definitive causal relationships. Although we found a significant correlation between anemia and SF in the basal ganglia and thalamus. Miao et al. have shown an increase in deoxyhaemoglobin levels in hypoxic regions in anaemic patients, and this may even play a role in determining CFS [112]. The exact physiological and pathological mechanism responsible for this connection has not yet been definitively established. Although we found that diabetes is significantly associated with CFS and that its occurrence is more likely in men, we had anticipated that male gender would be a risk factor, but found that women were more likely to have CFS. Even after adjusting for the onset of diabetes as an initial clinical sign or at follow-up, men also remained negatively associated with CFS. The literature has raised debates about gender-specific FS. In patients with Alzheimer's or

Parkinson's disease, research has shown that CFS is higher in men than in women. However, several studies have shown that women accumulate more iron in the brain than men, even when the HFE gene is mutated [112-114]. This suggested that women's brains may be more sensitive to iron deficiency than men's, leading to more CFS [112-114].

According to our data, while only abnormal movements were associated with FS in the putamen and pallidum, and cognitive impairment with FS in the cerebral cortex, there were no other statistically significant associations between NP symptoms and FS. The influence of CFS on the emergence of NP symptoms cannot be ruled out. We therefore propose to consider alternative hypotheses. We noted that people with epileptic seizures had significantly lower blood glucose levels than those without. This suggests a potential association between hypoglycemia and the onset of these seizures, rather than CFS. Furthermore, insulin has been shown to enhance memory by regulating synaptic plasticity in the hippocampus [115], so insulin resistance in PCA may lead to cognitive impairment. Furthermore, research has demonstrated a marked reduction in dopamine synthesis within striatal synaptosomes in diabetic rats compared with the control group [115]. Consequently, we can suggest that parkinsonism could also be attributed to insulin resistance and impaired glucose metabolism. Based on these findings, we can suggest that in addition to CFS, NP symptoms may also be induced by metabolic disturbances resulting from diabetes and anemia in PCA. While the reasons why patients with extremely low CP levels start the disease with systemic symptoms and later develop NP symptoms and CFS are evident in our data, the pathophysiological link between a moderate decrease in CP levels and disease initiation with NP signs, particularly in patients with normal brain MRI, remains unclear. The normal conventional MRI may be explained by a small amount of iron deposition that cannot be detected by conventional brain MRI. This hypothesis has been supported by case reports in which patients without CFS started with NP symptoms, while pathological analysis showed mild CFS in the basal ganglia and thalamus, with a slight decrease in neuron number and significant depletion of Purkinje cells the cerebellar cortex [30].

Our meta-analysis was limited by the number of published cases of this rare disease. Furthermore, published studies did not always include all data, such as biological results or brain MRI.

5. Conclusion

In this meta-analysis, we found that in the early stages of aceruloplasminemia, men tend to develop diabetes first, while women are more likely to suffer from anemia early on. Individuals under 50 are more likely to present with systemic signs, and those over 50 tend to present primarily with neuropsychiatric symptoms. Our results showed that several factors contribute to these varied phenotypes. Diabetes was the predominant factor associated with cerebral iron overload.

References

[1]   C.H. Ou-Yang, H.I. Lin, C.H. Lin, Generation of a human induced pluripotent stem cell line NTUHi002-A from a patient with aceruloplasminemia harboring a homozygous splicing mutation c.607+1 delG in CP gene, Stem Cell Res 63 (2022), 102856, https://doi.org/10.1016/j.scr.2022.102856.

[2]   N.E. Hellman, J.D. Gitlin, Ceruloplasmin metabolism and function, Annu. Rev. Nutr. 22 (2002) 439-458, https://doi.org/10.1146/annurev. nutr.22.012502.114457.

[3]   H. Miyajima, Aceruloplasminemia, Neuropathology 35 (2015) 83-90, https:// doi.org/10.1111/neup.12149.

[4]   M.J. Page, J.E. McKenzie, P.M. Bossuyt, I. Boutron, T.C. Hoffmann, C.D. Mulrow, L. Shamseer, J.M. Tetzlaff, E.A. Akl, S.E. Brennan, R. Chou, J. Glanville, J. M. Grimshaw, A. Hr'objartsson, M.M. Lalu, T. Li, E.W. Loder, E. Mayo-Wilson, S. McDonald, L.A. McGuinness, L.A. Stewart, J. Thomas, A.C. Tricco, V.A. Welch, P. Whiting, D. Moher, The PRISMA 2020 statement: an updated guideline for reporting systematic reviews, BMJ 372 (2021) n71, https://doi.org/10.1136/ bmj.n71.

[5]   Z. Miyake, K. Nakamagoe, K. Yoshida K, T. Kondo, A. Tamaoka, Deferasirox might be effective for microcytic anemia and neurological symptoms associated with aceruloplasminemia: a case report and review of the literature, Intern. Med. 59 (2020) 1755-1761.

[6]   A. McNeill, M. Pandolfo, J. Kuhn, H. Shang, H. Miyajima, The neurological presentation of ceruloplasmin gene mutations, Eur. Neurol. 60 (2008) 200-205, https://doi.org/10.1159/000148691.

[7]   C.M. Anugwom, C.G. Moscoso, N. Lim, M. Hassan, Aceruloplasminemia: a case report and review of a rare and misunderstood disorder of iron accumulation, Cureus 12 (2020), e11648, https://doi.org/10.7759/cureus.

[8]   L.H.P. Vroegindeweij, A.J.W. Boon, J.H.P. Wilson, J.G. Langendonk, Effects of iron chelation therapy on the clinical course of aceruloplasminemia: an analysis of aggregated case reports, Orphanet J. Rare Dis. 15 (2020) 105, https://doi. org/ 10.1186/s13023-020-01385.

[9]   M. Walterfang, E. March, D. Varghese, K. Miller, L. Simpson, B. Tomlinson, D. Velakoulis, Schizophrenia-like psychosis and aceruloplasminemia, Neuropsychiatr. Dis. Treat. 2 (2006) 577-581, https://doi.org/10.2147/ nedt.2006.2.4.577.

[10]   T. Kawanami, T. Kato, M. Daimon, M. Tominaga, H. Sasaki, K. Maeda, S. Arai, Y. Shikama, T. Katagiri, Hereditary caeruloplasmin deficiency: Clinicopathological study of a patient, J. Neurol. Neurosurg. Psychiatry 61 (1996) 506-509, https://doi.org/10.1136/jnnp.61.5.506.

[11]   Z.L. Harris, Y. Takahashi, H. Miyajima, M. Serizawa, R.T. MacGillivray, J. D. Gitlin, Aceruloplasminemia: molecular characterization of this disorder of iron metabolism, Proc. Natl. Acad. Sci. USA 92 (1995) 2539-2543, https://doi.org/ doi.org10.1073/pnas.92.7.2539.

[12]   S. Bosio, M. De Gobbi, A. Roetto, G. Zecchina, E. Leonardo, M. Rizzetto, C. Lucetti, L. Petrozzi, U.

Bonuccelli, C. Camaschella, Anemia and iron overload due to compound heterozygosity for novel ceruloplasmin mutations, Blood 100 (2002) 2246-2248, https://doi.org/10.1182/blood-2002-02-0584.

[13] M. Watanabe, C. Asai, K. Ishikawa, A. Kiyota, T. Terada, S. Kono, H. Miyajima, A. Okumura, Central diabetes insipidus and hypothalamic hypothyroidism associated with aceruloplasminemia, Intern Med 49 (2010) 1581-1585, https:// doi.org/10.2169/internalmedicine .49.3508.

[14] Y. Suzuki, K. Yoshida, Y. Aburakawa, K. Kuroda, T. Kimura, T. Terada, S. Kono, H. Miyajima, O. Yahara, Effectiveness of oral iron chelator treatment with deferasirox in an aceruloplasminemia patient with a novel ceruloplasmin gene mutation, Intern Med 52 (2013) 1527-1530, https://doi.org/10.2169/internalmedicine.52.0102.

[15] M. Kerkhof, P. Honkoop, Never forget aceruloplasminemia in case of highly suggestive Wilson's disease score, Hepatology 59 (2014) 1645-1647, https://doi. org/10.1002/hep.26719 (n.d).

[16] M. Ogimoto, K. Anzai, H. Takenoshita, K. Kogawa, Y. Akehi, R. Yoshida, M. Nakano, K. Yoshida, J. Ono, Criteria for early identification of aceruloplasminemia, Intern Med 50 (2011) 1415-1418, https://doi.org/10.2169/internalmedicine. 50.5108.

[17] Y. Hatanaka, T. Okano, K. Oda, K. Yamamoto, K. Yoshida, Aceruloplasminemia with juvenile-onset diabetes mellitus caused by exon skipping in the ceruloplasmin gene, Intern Med 42 (2003) 599-604, https://doi.org/10.2169/ internalmedicine .42.599.

[18] N.E. Hellman, M. Schaefer, S. Gehrke, P. Stegen, W.J. Hoffman, J.D. Gitlin, W. Stremmel, Hepatic iron overload in aceruloplasminaemia, Gut 47 (2000) 858-860, https://doi.org/10.1136/gut.47.6.858.

[19] A. Meral Gunes, M. Sezgin Evim, B. Baytan, A. Iwata, A. Hida, R. Avci, Aceruloplasminemia in a Turkish adolescent with a novel mutation of ceruloplasmin gene: the first diagnosed case from Turkey, J. Pediatr. Hematol. Oncol. 36 (2014) 423-425, https://doi.org/10.1097/MPH.0000000000000053.

[20] C. Bethlehem, B. van Harten, M. Hoogendoorn, Central nervous system involvement in a rare genetic iron overload disorder, Neth. J. Med 68 (2010) 316-318.

[21] M. Daimon, S. Susa, T. Ohizumi, S. Moriai, T. Kawanami, A. Hirata, H. Yamaguchi, H. Ohnuma, M. Igarashi, T. Kato, A novel mutation of the ceruloplasmin gene in a patient with heteroallelic ceruloplasmin gene mutation (HypoCPGM), Tohoku J. Exp. Med 191 (2000) 119-125, https://doi.org/ 10.1620/tjem.191.119.

[22] H. Lobbes, Q. Reynaud, S. Mainbourg, C. Savy-Stortz, M. Ropert, E. Bardou- Jacquet, S. Durupt, A new pathogenic missense variant in a consanguineous north-african family responsible for a highly variable aceruloplasminemia phenotype: a case-report, Front Neurosci. 16 (2022), 906360, https://doi.org/ 10.3389/fnins.2022.906360.

[23] M. Hayashida, S. Hashioka, H. Miki, M. Nagahama, R. Wake, T. Miyaoka, J. Horiguchi, Aceruloplasminemia with psychomotor excitement and neurological sign was improved by minocycline (Case

Report), Med. (Baltim.) 95 (2016), e3594, https://doi.org/10.1097/MD.0000000000003594.

[24] H. Miyajima, Y. Takahashi, H. Shimizu, N. Sakai, T. Kamata, E. Kaneko, Late onset diabetes mellitus in patients
with hereditary aceruloplasminemia, Intern Med 35 (1996) 641-645,
https://doi.org/10.2169/internalmedicine.35.641 (r. d).

[25] M. OndrejkovEcov'a, S. Dra^/ilov'a. M. Drakulov'a, J.L. Siles, R. Zemjarov'a Mezensk'a, P. Jungov'a, M. Fabi'an, B. Rychly, M. ^Zigrai. New mutation of the ceruloplasmin gene in the case of a neurologically asymptomatic patient with microcytic anaemia, obesity and supposed Wilson's disease, BMC Gastroenterol. 20 (2020), 95, https://doi.org/10.1186/s12876-020-0_237-8.

[26] A. Matsushima, T. Yoshida, K. Yoshida, S. Ohara, Y. Toyoshima, A. Kakita, S. Ikeda, Superficial siderosis associated with aceruloplasminemia. Case report, J. Neurol. Sci. 339 (2014) 231-234,
https://doi.org/10.1016/j.jns.2014.02.014.

[27] O. Furashova, S. Mielke, U. Lindner, Asymptomatic ocular manifestations of aceruloplasminemia in two adult white siblings: a multimodal imaging approach, Retin Cases Brief. Rep. 17 (2023) 273-278.

[28] M. Grisoli, A. Piperno, L. Chiapparini, R. Mariani, M. Savoiardo, MR imaging of cerebral cortical involvement in aceruloplasminemia, AJNR Am. J. Neuroradiol. 26 (2005) 657-661.

[29] S.T. Aydemir, O. Bulut, S. Ceylaner, M.C. Akbostanci, Aceruloplasminemia presenting with asymmetric chorea due to a novel frameshift mutation, Mov. Disord. Clin. Pr. 7 (2020) S67-S70, https://doi.org/10.1002/mdc3.13062.
[30] H. Miyajima, S. Kono, Y. Takahashi, M. Sugimoto, M. Sakamoto, N. Sakai, Cerebellar ataxia associated with
heteroallelic ceruloplasmin gene mutation, Neurology 57 (2001) 2205-2210,
https://doi.org/10.1212/wnl.57.12.2205.

[31] S. Nagata, N. Ikegaya, S. Ogino, S. Uchida, M. Itaya, A. Momita, S. Shinozaki, M. Ohura, K. Kuriki, S. Kono, H. Miyajima, A. Hishida, The resection of thyroid cancer was associated with the resolution of hyporesponsiveness to an erythropoiesis-stimulating agent in a hemodialysis patient with aceruloplasminemia, Intern Med 56 (2017) 805810, https://doi.org/10.2169/ internalmedicine.56.7455.

[32] M.H. Bjork, I.O. Gjerde, C. Tzoulis, R.J. Ulvik, L.A. Bindoff, A man in his 50s with high ferritin levels and increasing cognitive impairment (English, Norwegian), Tidsskr. Nor. Laege 135 (2015) 1369-1372, https://doi.org/10.4045/ tidsskr. 14.1115.

[33] I. Haemers, S. Kono, S. Goldman, J.D. Gitlin, M. Pandolfo, Clinical, molecular, and PET study of a case of aceruloplasminaemia presenting with focal cranial dyskinesia, J. Neurol. Neurosurg. Psychiatry 75 (2004) 334-337, https://doi.org/ 10.1136/jnnp.2003.017434.

[34] M. Badat, B. Kaya, P. Telfer, Combination-therapy with concurrent deferoxamine and deferiprone is

effective in treating resistant cardiac iron-loading in aceruloplasminaemia, Br. J. Haematol. 171 (2015) 430-432, https://doi.org/ 10.1111/bjh.13401.

[35] Y. Takeuchi, M. Yoshikawa, T. Tsujino, S. Kohno, N. Tsukamoto, A. Shiroi, E. Kikuchi, H. Fukui, H. Miyajima, A case of aceruloplasminaemia: abnormal serum ceruloplasmin protein without ferroxidase activity, J. Neurol. Neurosurg. Psychiatry 72 (2002) 543-545, https://doi.org/10.1136/jnnp.72.4.543.

[36] F. Chr'etien, J. Servan, J. Mikol, M. Trierweiller, D. Elghozi, F. Gray, A 70-year-old man with extrapyramidal symptoms, dementia and hemosiderosis, Brain Pathol. 16 (2006) 235-236, https://doi.org/10.1111/j.1750- 3639.2006.00014 1.x.

[37] M. Yonekawa, T. Okabe, Y. Asamoto, M. Ohta, A case of hereditary ceruloplasmin deficiency with iron deposition in the brain associated with chorea, dementia, diabetes mellitus and retinal pigmentation: administration of fresh-frozen human plasma, Eur. Neurol. 42 (1999) 157-162, https://doi.org/10.1159/000008091.

[38] K. Yamaguchi, S. Takahashi, T. Kawanami, T. Kato, H. Sasaki, Retinal degeneration in hereditary ceruloplasmin deficiency, Ophthalmologica 212 (1998) 11-14, https://doi.org/10.1159/000027251.

[39] H.F. Shang, X.F. Jiang, J.M. Burgunder, Q. Chen, D. Zhou, Novel mutation in the ceruloplasmin gene causing a cognitive and movement disorder with diabetes mellitus, Mov. Disord. 21 (2006) 2217-2220, https://doi.org/10.1002/ mds.21121.

[40] M. Rusticeanu, V. Zimmer, L. Schleithoff, K. Wonney, J. Viera, A. Zimmer, U. Hübschen, R.M. Bohle, F. Grünhage, F. Lammert, Novel ceruloplasmin mutation causing aceruloplasminemia with hepatic iron overload and diabetes without neurological symptoms, Clin. Genet 85 (2014) 300-301, https://doi.org/ 10.1111/cge.12145.

[41] Y. Xiao, C. Zhu, F. Jiang, Q. Gao, H. Lu H, C. Wang, L. Wei, Novel ceruloplasmin gene mutation causing aceruloplasminemia with diabetes in a Chinese woman: a case report, Ann. Palliat. Med 11 (2022) 2516-2522, https://doi.org/10.21037/ apm-21-1086.

[42] C.C. Ronquillo, L. Sauer, D. Morgan, J.B. Heckzo, D.J. Creel, N. Mamalis, M. M. DeAngelis, G.S. Hagemann, P.S. Bernstein, Absence of macular degeneration in a patient with aceruloplasminemia, Retina 39 (2019) 1824-1828, https://doi. org/10.1097/IAE.0000000000002628.

[43] R. Roberti Mdo, H.M. Borges Filho, C.H. Gonçalves, F.L. Lima, Aceruloplasminemia: a rare disease - diagnosis and treatment of two cases, Rev. Bras. Hematol. Hemoter. 33 (2011) 389-392, https://doi.org/10.5581/1516- 8484.20110104.

[44] L. Poli, A. Alberici, P. Buzzi, E. Marchina, A. Lanari, C. Arosio, A. Ciccone, F. Semeraro, R. Gasparotti, A. Padovani, B. Borroni, Is aceruloplasminemia treatable? Combining iron chelation and fresh-frozen plasma treatment, Neurol. Sci. 38 (2017) 357-360, https://doi.org/10.1007/s10072-016-2756-x.

[45] F. P'erez-Aguilar, J.A. Burguera, S. Benlloch, M. Berenguer, J.M. Ray'on, Aceruloplasminemia in an

asymptomatic patient with a new mutation. Diagnosis and family genetic analysis, J. Hepatol. 42 (2005) 947-949, https://doi.org/ 10.1016/j.jhep.2005.02.013.

[46] S. Pelucchi, R. Mariani, G. Ravasi, I. Pelloni, M. Marano, L. Tremolizzo, M. Alessio, A. Piperno, Phenotypic heterogeneity in seven Italian cases of aceruloplasminemia, Park. Relat. Disord. 51 (2018) 36-42, https://doi.org/ 10.1016/j.parkreldis.2018.02.036.

[47] N.E. Parks, R.A. Vandorpe, J.J. Moeller, Teaching NeuroImages: neurodegeneration with brain iron accumulation in aceruloplasminemia, Neurology 81 (2013) e151-e152, https://doi.org/10.1212/01. wnl.0000435557.21319.ad.

[48] H. Morita, S. Ikeda, K. Yamamoto, S. Morita, K. Yoshida, S. Nomoto, M. Kato, N. Yanagisawa, Hereditary ceruloplasmin deficiency with hemosiderosis: a clinicopathological study of a Japanese family, Ann. Neurol. 37 (1995) 646-656, https://doi.org/10.1002/ana.410370515.

[49] J.L. Dunaief, C. Richa, E.P. Franks, R.L. Schultze, T.S. Aleman, J.F. Schenck, E. A. Zimmerman, D.G. Brooks, Macular degeneration in a patient with aceruloplasminemia, a disease associated with retinal iron overload, Ophthalmology 112 (2005) 1062-1065, https://doi.org/10.1016/]. ophtha.2004.12.029.

[50] D. Di Raimondo, A. Pinto, A. Tuttolomondo, P. Fernandez, C. Camaschella, G. Licata, Aceruloplasminemia: a case report, Intern Emerg. Med. 3 (2008) 395-399, https://doi.org/10.1007/s11739-008-0150-2.

[51] R. Muroi, H. Yagyu, H. Kobayashi, M. Nagata, N. Sato, J. Ideno, N. Fujita, A. Ando, K. Okada, Y. Takiyama, S. Nagasaka, H. Miyajima, I. Nakano, S. Ishibashi, Early onset insulin-dependent diabetes mellitus as an initial manifestation of aceruloplasminaemia, Diabet. Med. 23 (2006) 1136-1139, https://doi.org/10.1111/j.1464- 5491.2006.01883.x.

[52] M. Watanabe, K. Ohyama, M. Suzuki, Y. Nosaki, T. Hara, K. Iwai, S. Kono, H. Miyajima, K. Mokuno, Aceruloplasminemia with abnormal compound heterozygous mutations developed neurological dysfunction during phlebotomy therapy, Intern. Med. 15 (2018) 2713-2718, https://doi.org/10.2169/ internalmedicine.9855-17.

[53] H. Miyajima, Y. Takahashi, S. Kono, A Hishida, K. Ishikawa, M. Sakamoto, Frontal lobe dysfunction associated with glucose hypometabolism in aceruloplasminemia, J. Neurol. 252 (2005) 996-997, https://doi.org/10.1007/ s00415-005-0796-x.

[54] H. Miyajima, Y. Takahashi, M. Serizawa, E. Kaneko, J.D. Gitlin, Increased plasma lipid peroxidation in patients with aceruloplasminemia, Free Radic. Biol. Med. 20 (1996) 757-760, https://doi.org/10.1016/0891-5849(95)02178- 7.

[55] J.M. Melgari, M. Marano, C.C. Quattrocchi, A. Piperno, C. Arosio, M. Frontali, S. Nuovo, M. Siotto, G. Salomone, R. Altavilla, L. di Biase, F. Scrascia, R. Squitti, F. Vernieri, Movement disorders and brain iron overload in a new subtype of aceruloplasminemia, Park. Relat. Disord. 21 (2015) 658-660, https://doi.org/

10.1016/j.parkreldis.2015.03.014.

[56] O. Lor'eal, B. Turlin, C. Pigeon, A. Moisan, M. Ropert, P. Morice, Y. Gandon, A. M. Jouanolle, M. V'erin, R.C. Hider, K. Yoshida, P. Brissot, Aceruloplasminemia: new clinical, pathophysiological and therapeutic insights, J. Hepatol. 36 (6) (2002) 851, https://doi.org/10.1016/s0168-8278(02)00042-9.

[57] U. Lindner, D. Schuppan, L. Schleithoff, J.O. Habeck, T. Grodde, K. Kirchhof, U. Stoelzel, Aceruloplasminaemia: a family with a novel mutation and long-term therapy with deferasirox, Horm. Metab. Res 47 (2015) 303-308, https://doi.org/ 10.1055/s-0034-1383650.

[58] M.C. Hines, Hl Bonkovsky, S.R. Rudnick, J.T. Mhoon, Peripheral neuropathy and the ceruloplasmin gene, Ann. Intern 168 (2018) 894-895, https://doi.org/ 10.7326/L17-0621.

[59] A. Hida, H. Kowa, A. Iwata, M. Tanaka, S. Kwak, S. Tsuji, Aceruloplasminemia in a Japanese woman with a novel mutation of CP gene: clinical presentations and analysis of genetic and molecular pathogenesis, J. Neurol. Sci. 298 (2010) 136-139, https://doi.org/10.1016/j.ins.2010.08.019.

[60] J. Kuhn, H. Miyajima, Y. Takahashi, B. Kunath, U. Hartmann-Klosterkoetter, D. Cooper- Mahkorn, M. Schaefer, H. Bewermeyer, Extrapyramidal and cerebellar movement disorder in association with heterozygous ceruloplasmin gene mutation, J. Neurol. 252 (2005) 111-113, https://doi.org/10.1007/s00415-005- 0608-3.

[61] J. Kuhn, H. Bewermeyer, H. Miyajima, Y. Takahashi, K.F. Kuhn, T. U. Hoogenraad, Treatment of symptomatic heterozygous aceruloplasminemia with oral zinc sulphate, Brain Dev. 29 (2007) 450-453, https://doi.org/10.1016/ j.braindev.2007.01.001.

[62] S. Kono, H. Suzuki, K. Takahashi, Y. Takahashi, K. Shirakawa, Y. Murakawa, S. Yamaguchi, H. Miyajima, Hepatic iron overload associated with a decreased serum ceruloplasmin level in a novel clinical type of aceruloplasminemia, Gastroenterology 131 (2006) 240-245, https://doi.org/10.1053/j. gastro.2006.04.017.

[63] A. Finkenstedt, E. Wolf, E. Hofner, B.I. Gasser, S. B "osch. R. Bakry, M. Creus, C. Kremser, M. Schocke, M. Theurl, P. Moser, M. Schranz, G. Bonn, W. Poewe, W. Vogel, A.R. Janecke, H. Zoller, Hepatic but not brain iron is rapidly chelated by deferasirox in aceruloplasminemia due to a novel gene mutation, J. Hepatol. 53 (2010) 1101- 1107, https://doi.org/10.1016/j.jhep.2010.04.039.

[64] S. Kohno, H. Miyajima, Y. Takahashi, Y. Inoue, Aceruloplasminemia with a novel mutation associated with parkinsonism, Neurogenetics 2 (2000) 237-238, https://doi.org/10.1007/s100489900082.

[65] H.K. Kim, C.S. Ki, Y.J. Kim, M.S. Lee, Radiological Findings of Two Sisters with Aceruloplasminemia Presenting with Chorea, Clin. Neuroradiol. 27 (2017) 385-388, https://doi.org/10.1007/s00062-017-0573-0.

[66] R. Kassubek, I. Uttner, C. Schonfeldt-Lecuona, J. Kassubek, B.J. Connemann, Extending the aceruloplasminemia phenotype: NBIA on imaging and acanthocytosis, yet only minor neurological findings, J. Neurol. Sci. 376 (2017) 151-152, https://doi.org/10.1016/j.ins.2017.03.019.

[67] A. Jim'enez-Huete, J. Bernar, H. Miyajima, Y. Takahashi, J. Alvarez-Linera, O. Franch, M.S. van der

Knaap, Multiple motor system dysfunction associated with a heterozygous ceruloplasmin gene mutation, J. Neurol. 255 (2008) 1083-1084, https://doi.org/10.1007/s00415- 008-0823-9.

[68] W.P. Hofmann, C. Welsch, Y. Takahashi, H. Miyajima, U. Mihm, C. Krick, S. Zeuzem, C. Sarrazin, Identification and in silico characterization of a novel compound heterozygosity associated with hereditary aceruloplasminemia, Scand. J. Gastroenterol. 42 (2007) 1088-1094, https://doi.org/10.1080/ 00365520701278810.

[69] A. Fasano, C. Colosimo, H. Miyajima, P.A. Tonali, T.J. Re, A.R. Bentivoglio, Aceruloplasminemia: a novel mutation in a family with marked phenotypic variability, Mov. Disord. 23 (2008) 751-755, https://doi.org/10.1002/ mds.21938.

[70] M. Daimon, T. Kato, T. Kawanami, M. Tominaga, M. Igarashi, K. Yamatani, H. Sasaki, A nonsense mutation of the ceruloplasmin gene in hereditary ceruloplasmin deficiency with diabetes mellitus, Biochem Biophys. Res Commun. 217 (1995) 89-95, https://doi.org/10.1006/bbrc.1995.2749.

[71] M. Tai, N. Matsuhashi, O. Ichii, T. Suzuki, Y. Ejiri, S. Kono, T. Terada, H. Miyajima, M. Harada, Case of presymptomatic aceruloplasminemia treated with deferasirox, Hepatol. Res 44 (2014) 1253-1258, https://doi.org/10.1111/ hepr.12292.

[72] Y. Takahashi, H. Miyajima, S. Shirabe, S. Nagataki, A. Suenaga, J.D. Gitlin, Characterization of a nonsense mutation in the ceruloplasmin gene resulting in diabetes and neurodegenerative disease, Hum. Mol. Genet 5 (1996) 81-84, https://doi.org/10.1093/hmg/5.1.81.

[73] P. Feraco, A. Conficoni, B. Petralia, P. Lanza, Brain iron accumulation: don't forget aceruloplasminemia, Eur. Biomed. 15 (2020) 107-109.

[74] F. Touarsa, D.A. Mohamed, B. Onka, S. Rostoum, N. Ech-Cherif El Kettani, M. Fikri, M. Jiddane, Brain iron accumulation on MRI revealing aceruloplasminemia: a rare cause of simultaneous brain and systemic iron overload, BJR Case Rep. 8 (2022) 20220035, https://doi.org/10.1259/ bjrcr.20220035.

[75] J.I. Logan, K.B. Harveyson, G.B. Wisdom, A.E. Hughes, G.P. Archbold, Hereditary caeruloplasmin deficiency, dementia and diabetes mellitus, QJM 87 (1994) 663-670.

[76] N. Okamoto, S. Wada, T. Oga, Y. Kawabata, Y. Baba, D. Habu, Z. Takeda, Y. Wada, Hereditary ceruloplasmin deficiency with hemosiderosis, Hum. Genet 97 (1996) 755-758, https://doi.org/10.1007/BF02346185.

[77] G. Ravasi, S. Pelucchi, F. Canonico, R. Mariani, A. Piperno, Atypical phenotype in a patient with ceruloplasmin
mutations in the compound heterozygous state, Meta Gene 29 (2021), 100905, https://doi.org/10.1016/j.mgene.2021.100905.

[78] L. Zhou, Y. Chen, Y. Li, S. Gharabaghi, Y. Chen, S.K. Sethi, Y. Wu, E.M. Haacke, Intracranial iron

distribution and quantification in aceruloplasminemia: A case study, Magn. Reson Imaging 70 (2020) 29-35, https://doi.org/10.1016/]. mri.2020.02.016.

[79]   F.M. Skidmore, V. Drago, P. Foster, I.M. Schmalfuss, K.M. Heilman, R.R. Streiff, Aceruloplasminaemia with progressive atrophy without brain iron overload: treatment with oral chelation, J. Neurol. Neurosurg. Psychiatry 79 (2008) 467-470, https://doi.org/10.1136/]nnp.2007.120568.

[80]   Y. Arslan, U. S_j ener, A. Sariteke, Y. Zorlu, Aceruloplasminemia presenting with cognitive impairment, Turk. J. Neurol. 23 (2017) 134-135, https://doi.org/ 10.4274/tnd.37640.

[81]   R. Mariani, C. Arosio, S. Pelucchi, M. Grisoli, A. Piga, P. Trombini, A. Piperno, Iron chelation therapy in aceruloplasminaemia: study of a patient with a novel missense mutation, Gut 53 (2004) 756-758, https://doi.org/10.1136/ gut.2003.030429.

[82]   G.L. Calder, M.H. Lee, N. Sachithanandan, S. Bell, H. Zeimer, R.J. MacIsaac, Aceruloplasminaemia: a disorder of diabetes and neurodegeneration, Intern Med J. 47 (2017) 115-118, https://doi.org/10.1111/imj.13309.

[83]   G.M. Riboldi, K. Anstett, R. Jain, H. Lau, D. Swope, Aceruloplasminemia and putaminal cavitation, Park. Relat. Disord. 51 (2018) 121-123, https://doi.org/ 10.1016/j.parkreldis.2018.03.003.

[84]   B. Park, E.A. Yoo, H.S. Park, Aceruloplasminemia presents as type 2 diabetes associated with unexplained microcytic anemia: a case report, J. Korean. Diabetes 23 (2022) 144-152, https://doi.org/10.4093/jkd.2022.23.2.144.

[85]   F. Ashrafi, M. Salari, F. Nouri, F. Shiravi, Dementia as a core clinical feature of a patient with aceruloplasminemia, Clin. Case Rep. 10 (2022), e05581, https://doi. org/10.1002/ccr3.5581.

[86]   A. Yamamura, Y. Kikukawa, K. Tokunaga, E. Miyagawa, S. Endo, H. Miyake, H. Hata, H. Mitsuya, K. Yoshida, M. Matsuoka, Pancytopenia and myelodysplastic changes in aceruloplasminemia: a case with a novel pathogenic variant in the ceruloplasmin gene, Intern Med 57 (2018) 1905-1910, https://doi.org/10.2169/ internalmedicine.9496- 17.

[87]   M. Watanabe, K. Ohyama, M. Suzuki, Y. Nosaki, T. Hara, K. Iwai, S. Kono, H. Miyajima, K. Mokuno, Aceruloplasminemia with abnormal compound heterozygous mutations developed neurological dysfunction during phlebotomy therapy, Intern Med 57 (2018) 2713-2718, https://doi.org/10.2169/ internalmedicine.9855-17.

[88]   F. Ashrafi, M. Salari, F. Nouri, F. Shiravi, Dementia as a core clinical feature of a patient with aceruloplasminemia, Clin. Case Rep. 10 (2022), e05581, https://doi. org/10.1002/ccr3.5581.

[89]   A. Doyle, F. Rusli, P. Bhathal, Aceruloplasminaemia: a rare but important cause of iron overload, bcr2014207541, BMJ Case Rep. 2015 (2015), https://doi.org/ 10.1136/bcr-2014-207541.

[90]   G. Marchi, F. Busti F, A.L. Zidanes, A. Castagna, D. Girelli, Aceruloplasminemia: a severe neurodegenerative disorder deserving an early diagnosis, Front. Neurosci. 13 (2019), 325,

https://doi.org/10.3389/fnins.2019.00325.

[91] L.H.P. Vroegindeweij, E.H. van der Beek, A.J.W. Boon, M. Hoogendoorn, J. A. Kievit, J.H.P. Wilson, J.G. Langendonk, Aceruloplasminemia presents as Type 1 diabetes in non-obese adults: a detailed case series, Diabet. Med. 32 (2015) 993-1000, https://doi.org/10.11.

[92] H. Miyajima, Y. Hosoi, Aceruloplasminemia, In: MP. Adam, GM. Mirzaa, RA. Pagon, SE. Wallace, LJH. Bean, KW. Gripp, A. Amemiya A (Eds), GeneReviews® [Internet], Seattle (WA): University of Washington, Seattle; 1993-2023.

[93] M. Vila Cuenca, G. Marchi, A. Barqu'e, C. Esteban-Jurado, A. Marchetto, A. Giorgetti, V. Chelban, H. Houlden, N.W. Wood, C. Piubelli, M. Dorigatti Borges, D. Martins de Albuquerque, K. Yotsumoto Fertrin, E. Jov'e- Buxeda, J. Sanchez-Delgado, N. Baena-Diez, B. Burnyte B, A. Utkus, F. Busti, G. Kaubrys, E. Suku, K. Kowalczyk, B. Karaszewski, J.B. Porter, S. Pollard, P. Eleftheriou, P. Bignell, D. Girelli, M. Sanchez, Genetic and clinical heterogeneity in thirteen new cases with aceruloplasminemia. atypical anemia as a clue for an early diagnosis, Int. J. Mol. Sci. 21 (2020) 2374, https://doi.org/10.3390/ ijms21072374.

[94] B.M.L. Stelten, W. van Ommen, K. Keizer, Neurodegeneration with brain iron accumulation: a novel mutation in the ceruloplasmin gene, JAMA Neurol. 76 (2019) 229-230, https://doi.org/10.1001/iamaneurol.2018.3230.

[95] X. Xu, S. Pin, M. Gathinji, R. Fuchs, Z.L. Harris, Aceruloplasminemia: an inherited neurodegenerative disease with impairment of iron homeostasis, Ann. N. Y. Acad. Sci. 1012 (2004) 299-305, https://doi.org/10.1196/annals. 1306.024.

[96] S. Chitturi, J. George, Interaction of iron, insulin resistance, and nonalcoholic steatohepatitis, Curr. Gastroenterol. Rep. 5 (2003) 18-25, https://doi.org/ 10.1007/s11894-003-0005-y.

[97] E. Arner, A.R. Forrest, A. Ehrlund, N. Mejhert, M. Itoh, H. Kawaji, T. Lassmann, J. Laurencikiene, M. Ryd'en, P. Arner, Ceruloplasmin is a novel adipokine which is overexpressed in adipose tissue of obese subjects and in obesity-associated cancer cells, PLoS One 9 (2014), e80274, https://doi.org/10.1371/journal. pone. 0080274.

[98] V.K. Sharma, A. Tumbapo, V. Pant, B. Aryal, S. Shrestha, B.K. Yadav, E. T. Tuladhar, A. Bhattarai, M. Rau, Ceruloplasmin, a potential marker for glycemic status and its relationship with lipid profile in Type II diabetes mellitus, Asian J. Med. Sci. 9 (2018) 3. https://doi.org/10.3126/ajms.v9i2.19003.

[99] Y. Sakuma, J. Ogino, R. Iwai, T. Inoue, H. Takahashi, Y. Suzuki, D. Kinoshita, K. Takemura, H. Takahashi, H. Shimura, Y. Sato, S. Yoshida, N. Hashimoto N, Hyperferritinemia is a predictor of onset of diabetes in japanese males independently of decreased renal function and fatty liver: a fifteen-year follow-up study, J. Clin. Med. Res. 13 (2021) 541-548, https://doi.org/10.14740/ jocmr4635.

[100] A. Aregbesola, S. Voutilainen, J.K. Virtanen, J. Mursu, T.P. Tuomainen, Body iron stores and the risk of type 2 diabetes in middle-aged men, Eur. J. Endocrinol. 169 (2013) 247-253, https://doi.org/10.1530/EJE-13-0145.

[101] S. Akter, A. Nanri, K. Kuwahara, Y. Matsushita, T. Nakagawa, M. Konishi, T. Honda T, S. Yamamoto, T. Hayashi, M. Noda, T. Mizoue, Circulating ferritin concentrations and risk of type 2 diabetes in Japanese individuals, J. Diabetes Invest. 8 (2017), 462-47.

[102] L. Zhidong, W. Miao, Z. Chunbo, Z. Shigao, J. Guang, Molecular functions of ceruloplasmin in metabolic disease pathology, Dovepress 15 (2022) 695-711, https://doi.org/10.2147/DMSO.S346648.

[103] R.C. Cooksey, H.A. Jouihan, R.S. Ajioka, M.W. Hazel, D.L. Jones, J.P. Kushner, D. A. McClain, Oxidative stress, beta-cell apoptosis, and decreased insulin secretory capacity in mouse models of hemochromatosis, Endocrinology 145 (2004) 5305-5312, https://doi.org/1

[104] F. Luan, Y. Chen, Y. Xu, X. Jiang, B. Liu, Y. Wang, Associations between whole blood trace elements concentrations and HbA1c levels in patients with type 2 diabetes, Biometals 35 (2022) 1011-1022, https://doi.org/10.1007/s10534-022- 00419-z.

[105] H. Noha, M. Maha, F. Laila, Trace elements and their relation to diabetes mellitus and obesity, JRAM 2 (2021) 128-132, https://doi.org/10.21608/ jram.2020.46094.1093.

[106] A.K. Jeppu, K.A. Kumar, A. Augusthy, Plasma glucose and serum ceruloplasmin in metabolic syndrome and diabetes mellitus type 2, Recent Adv. Biol. Med 2 (2016) 651, https://doi.org/10.18639/RABM.2016.02.282945.

[107] E.L. Harris, C.E. McLaren, D.M. Reboussin, V.R. Gordeuk, J.C. Barton, R.T. Acton, G.D. McLaren, T.M. Vogt, B.M. Snively, C. Leiendecker-Foster, J.L. Holup, L. V. Passmore, J.H. Eckfeldt, E. Lin, P.C. Adams, Serum ferritin and transferrin saturation in Asians and Pacific Islanders, Arch. Intern. Med. 167 (2007) 722-726, https://doi.org/10.1001/archinte.167.7.722.

[108] A. Al-Naseem, A. Sallam, S. Choudhury, J. Thachi, Iron deficiency without anaemia: a diagnosis that matters, Clin. Med 21 (2021) 107-111, https://doi.org/ 10.7861/clinmed.2020-0582.

[109] S. Raia, A. Conti, A. Zanardi, B. Ferrini, G.M. Scotti, E. Gilberti, G.D. Palma, S. David, M. Alessio, Ceruloplasmin-deficient mice show dysregulation of lipid metabolism in liver and adipose tissue reduced by a protein replacement, Int. J. Mol. Sci. 24 (2023) 1150, https://doi.org/10.3390/iims24021150.

[110] E. Corradini, E. Buzzetti, P. Dongiovanni, S. Scarlini, A. Caleffi, S. Pelusi, I. Bernardis, P. Ventura, R. Rametta, E. Tenedini, E. Tagliafico, A.L. Fracanzani, S. Fargion, A. Pietrangelo, L.V. Valenti, Ceruloplasmin gene variants are associated with hyperferritinemia and increased liver iron in patients with NAFLD, J. Hepatol. 75 (2021) 506-513, https://doi.org/10.1016/j. jhep.2021.03.014.

[111] J. Li, Q. Zhang, N. Zhang, L. Guo, Increased brain iron detection by voxel-based quantitative susceptibility mapping in type 2 diabetes mellitus patients with an executive function decline, Front. Neurosci. 14 (2021), 606182, https://doi.org/ 10.3389/fnins.

[112] X. Miao, S. Choi, B. Tamrazi, Y. Chai, C. Vu, T.D. Coates, J.C. Wood, Increased brain iron deposition in patients with sickle cell disease: an MRI quantitative susceptibility mapping study, Blood 132 (2018) 1618-

1621, https://doi.org/ 10.1182/blood-2018-04-8.

[113] N. Persson, J. Wu, Q. Zhang, T. Liu, J. Shen, R. Bao, M. Ni, T. Liu, Y. Wang, P. Spincemaille, Age and sex related differences in subcortical brain iron concentrations among healthy adults, Neuroimage 122 (2015) 385-398, https:// doi.org/10.1016/j.neuroimag.

[114] K.A. Duck, E.B. Neely, I.A. Simpson, J.R. Connor, A role for sex and a common HFE gene variant in brain iron uptake, J. Cereb. Blood Flow. Metab. 38 (2018) 540-548, https://doi.org/10.1177/0271678x17701949.

[115] E. Bl'azquez, V. Hurtado-Carneiro, Y. LeBaut-Ayuso, E. Vel'azquez, L. García- García, F. G'omez-Oliver, J.M. Ruiz-Albusac, J. 'Avila, M.A. Pozo, Significance of brain glucose hypometabolism, altered insulin signal transduction, and insulin resistance in several neurological diseases, Front Endocrinol. 13 (2022), 873301, https://doi.org/10.3389/fendo.2022.873301.

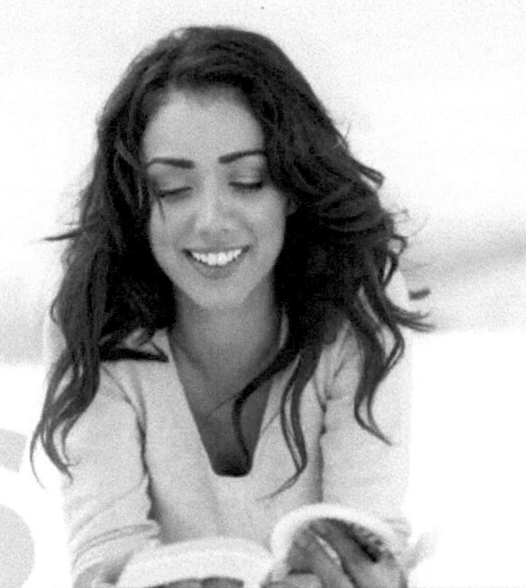

I want morebooks!

Buy your books fast and straightforward online - at one of world's fastest growing online book stores! Environmentally sound due to Print-on-Demand technologies.

Buy your books online at
www.morebooks.shop

Kaufen Sie Ihre Bücher schnell und unkompliziert online – auf einer der am schnellsten wachsenden Buchhandelsplattformen weltweit! Dank Print-On-Demand umwelt- und ressourcenschonend produziert.

Bücher schneller online kaufen
www.morebooks.shop

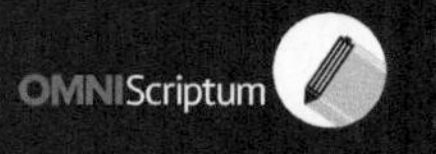

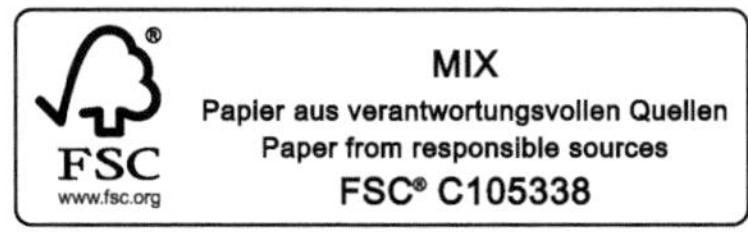

Printed by Books on Demand GmbH, Norderstedt / Germany